PALEO-
KETOGENIC
THE WHY AND THE HOW

Dedication

SM: To my lovely patients, who have been willing guinea pigs and most forgiving when my suggestions have not worked. However, in doing so, they have pushed forward the frontiers of Ecological Medicine.

CR: For Judith whom I have met once. On 15th March 1993, I walked out of Moorgate Place, my place of work, turned the corner into Copthall Avenue, and collapsed. This was the beginning of my ME and yes, it started on the Ides of March. I could not move my legs, I was confused, I had deafening tinnitus, I had all-over pain. The world was spinning. For around two hours, fellow City workers walked around me, even stepped over me, suspecting drunkenness or maybe that I was some kind of unusual, suited tramp. Then, this woman, about the same age as me at the time, 30 or so, stopped and bent down and sat on the pavement next to me. She listened to me. And believed me. She called a cab, got in the cab with me and got me to Paddington. She paid the cab. She then helped me, all wobbly, to get to a bench at the station. I had lost my season ticket, and much else in the confusion of the fall. She bought me a ticket for Oxford, and also a coffee, with lots of sugar, as I recall, and a croissant – not very PK, Judith! She waited with me until my train arrived, and made sure I got to a seat, and then I asked her who she was, and she gave me her business card, Judith….. I lost that business card in my confused state on the way home, and I have never been able to thank her. So, this is for you, Judith, thank you, and if you're out there and read this, I owe you a coffee.

PALEO-
KETOGENIC
THE WHY AND THE HOW

Just what *this* doctor ordered

Dr Sarah Myhill
and
Craig Robinson

Illustrations by Michelle McCullagh

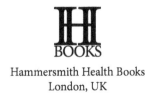

Hammersmith Health Books
London, UK

First published in 2022 by Hammersmith Health Books
– an imprint of Hammersmith Books Limited
4/4A Bloomsbury Square, London WC1A 2RP, UK
www.hammersmithbooks.co.uk

The information contained in this book is for educational purposes only. It is
the result of the study and the experience of the authors. Whilst the information
and advice offered are believed to be true and accurate at the time of going to
press, neither the authors nor the publisher can accept any legal responsibility or
liability for any errors or omissions that may have been made or for any adverse
effects which may occur as a result of following the recommendations given
herein. Always consult a qualified medical practitioner if you have any concerns
regarding your health.

British Library Cataloguing in Publication Data: A CIP record of this book is
available from the British Library.

Print ISBN 978-1-78161-217-0
Ebook ISBN 978-1-78161-218-7

Commissioning editor: Georgina Bentliff
Designed and typeset by: Julie Bennett of Bespoke Publishing Limited
Cover and inside illustrations: Michelle McCullagh
Cover design by: Madeline Meckiffe
Index: Dr Laurence Errington
Production: Deborah Wehner of Moatvale Press, UK
Printed and bound by: TJ Books Ltd, Cornwall, UK

Contents

Contents

Contents

Acknowledgements

We would like to thank the following for permission to reproduce their delicious recipes:
- Carolyn Chesshire
- Moira Creak
- Jason O'Sullivan
- Dee Marshall
- Christina Macleod
- Philippa Sherwood
- Mim Elkan
- Michelle McCullagh (and also for her wonderful illustrations)
- Sue McCullagh
- Wendy Cresswell
- Angie Jones
- Rosemary Segrott
- Dr Shideh Puria

About the Authors

Dr Sarah Myhill MB BS qualified in medicine (with Honours) from Middlesex Hospital Medical School in 1981 and has since focused tirelessly on identifying and treating the underlying causes of health problems, especially the 'diseases of civilisation' with which we are beset in the West. She has worked in the NHS and independent practice and for 17 years was the Honorary Secretary of the British Society for Ecological Medicine, which focuses on the causes of disease and treating through diet, supplements and avoiding toxic stress. She helps to run and lectures at the Society's training courses and also lectures regularly on organophosphate poisoning, the problems of silicone, and chronic fatigue syndrome. Visit her website at www.drmyhill.co.uk

Craig Robinson MA took a first in Mathematics at Oxford University in 1985. He then joined Price Waterhouse and qualified as a Chartered Accountant in 1988, after which he worked as a lecturer in the private sector, and also in the City of London, primarily in Financial Sector Regulation roles. Craig first met Sarah in 2001, as a patient for the treatment of his ME, and since then they have developed a professional working relationship, where he helps with the maintenance of www.drmyhill.co.uk, the moderating of Dr Myhill's Facebook groups and other ad hoc projects, as well as with the editing and writing of her books.

Stylistic note: Use of the first person singular in this book refers to me, Dr Sarah Myhill. One can assume that the medicine and biochemistry are mine, as edited by Craig Robinson and that the classical and mathematical references are Craig's.

Preface

Four decades of practical Naturopathic/Functional/Ecological medicine have taught me that the single most important intervention to prevent and treat disease is diet. Hardly surprising – we consume kilograms of food daily which, depending on content, has the potential to kill or cure. So what to eat?

With any such difficult question I always return to evolutionary principles. What is it that has allowed humans to survive the vicissitudes of a harsh and hostile world? How is it that *Homo sapiens* had the physical and mental strength not just to survive but to prevail over other species? To achieve such requires abundant energy and raw materials and the primary source of both is food. That diet which brought such evolutionary success is the paleo-ketogenic diet and is defined by those foods consumed for some hundreds of thousands of years and to which our body and brain have adapted so efficiently.

With modern securities of food supply, absence of predators, warmth and social safety, Humans should be the fittest and most able mammals on Earth? Not so – Westerners (and all those on a standard Western diet) are suffering epidemics of fatigue and obesity, degenerative disease and progressive pathology. Life expectancy is falling, we have more disabled people than ever and the intelligence of our children is declining. Why so? The single most important reason is again diet.

What went wrong? We now have access to a secure and better quality of food than ever before. The big issue is that we Westerners are addicts. Our lives are driven by addiction – from caffeine, nicotine and alcohol to smart phones and computer games. But the most overlooked, convenient, cheap but pernicious addiction is to sugar, fruit sugar, refined carbohydrates and starches. These foods are killing us.

Addictions seem wonderful because in the immediate short term they mask those deeply unpleasant symptoms of stress. In Lancashire chip shops, the chip butty emerged; in Ireland it was the sugar sandwich; and in Scotland, the deep-fried Mars Bar. These carbohydrate hits provided cheap, instant relief from fatigue, depression and anxiety. But this is ephemeral – you cannot have an upper without a downer. Such a downer could be alleviated by a further carbohydrate snack. Thus an addiction is born. Carbohydrates are consumed not for calorie needs but for symptom relief. The most stressed people become the fattest and the sickest.

The paleo-ketogenic diet is non-addictive. It further avoids evolutionary newcomers such as dairy products and gluten grains. It is the starting point to prevent and treat all disease. I spend more time talking about food and cooking than all other subjects put together. Hence our first PK Cookbook came into being. However, I soon found that just supplying a cookbook was not enough. I had also to deliver the intellectual imperatives to do the diet; the nitty gritty of calories, proteins, fats, fibres and ketones; together with anticipating the problems of the metabolic hinterland and diet, die-off and detox reactions. Readers were also clamouring for more examples of delicious recipes.

All who make this journey have a bumpy ride; some do not succeed at the first attempt; we all relapse on occasion. This book, *Paleo-Ketogenic: The Why and the How*, is born out of the experiences of hundreds of patients and their hundreds of questions, to deliver the most frictionless and painless route to success.

You must do a PK diet. Just do it.

Part I

The Why

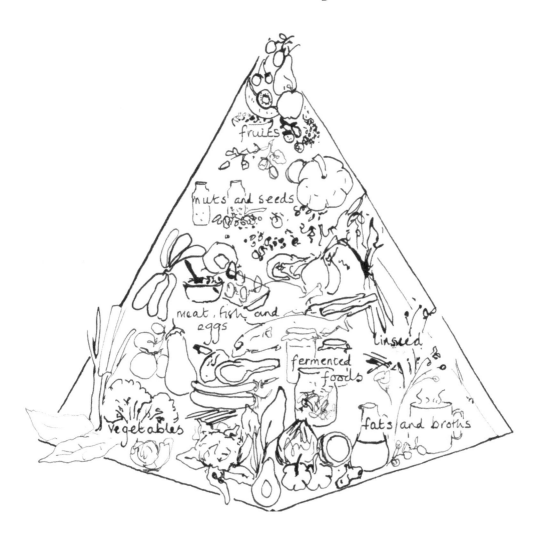

Chapter 1

Why we should all be eating a paleo-ketogenic (PK) diet

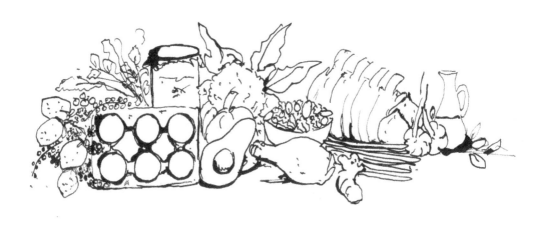

We should all be eating a paleo-ketogenic (PK) diet because this has been established by thousands of years of Evolution. This diet is also the starting point to prevent and treat all Western disease.

> *Let Medicine be thy food and food be thy medicine*
>   Hippocrates, c. 460 – c. 370 BC

Humans evolved over two and half million years eating a paleo-ketogenic diet. This is the diet which best suits our bowels, bodies and brains*. If we wish to live to our full potential in terms of quality and quantity of life, this is the diet naturally selected, by survival of the fittest, throughout Evolution.

Evolution is only really interested in getting us to childbearing age. Once Richard Dawkins's 'selfish gene'[1] has been passed on to the next generation, we are effectively on the evolutionary scrap heap. This means the survival strategies that get us to child-bearing age may be different from those that apply in older age. We should *all* be eating the PK diet *all* the time, but as we age, our bowels, bodies and brains work less efficiently and so the imperative to stick with this diet increases. Younger people can get away with less correct diets and this leads many to believe that their present diet is 'OK' because 'that is what I have always eaten'.

Primitive man gained huge evolutionary advantage through being able to run on two fuels – fats and carbohydrates. Indeed, we can eat a greater variety of foods than any other mammal (bar perhaps the pig – I love pigs!). This 'metabolic flexibility' plus the First Agricultural Revolution[†], around 10,000 BC, meant that more people survived, the land could support more of us and so more achieved child-bearing age than ever before.

The human population of Earth sky-rocketed with this 'dual fuel effect'. However, what gets us to child-bearing age is not necessarily good for optimum health and longevity. And the health of all, especially our precious children, is fast declining.

> *They [Young People] have exalted notions, because they have not been humbled by life or learned its necessary limitations; moreover, their hopeful disposition makes them think themselves equal to great things – and that means having exalted notions. They would always rather do noble deeds than useful ones. Their lives are regulated more by moral feeling than by reasoning – all their mistakes are in the direction of doing things excessively and vehemently. They overdo everything – they love too much, hate too much, and the same with everything else.*
>
> Aristotle, 384 – 322 BC

* Literary aside: The reader may have noticed that I have used both alliteration and the 'Rule of Three' when writing 'bowels, bodies and brains' as a literary technique to emphasise this point. The Rule of Three can be seen everywhere in famous speeches, such as 'Friends, Romans, Countrymen' and 'blood, sweat and tears', but it can also be seen in public safety campaigns: 'Stop, Look, Listen', 'Stay Home, Protect the NHS, Save Lives'; and in films too: 'The Good, the Bad and the Ugly'; and even when colonies decide they no longer wish to be colonies, as in 'Life, liberty and the pursuit of happiness'.

† Footnote: We're not talking Turnip Townsend and seed drills here – that was the second Agricultural Revolution.

Or, to quote Oscar Wilde: 'Youth is wasted on the young'.

Why ketogenic?

A ketogenic diet is healthy because it is low in carbohydrates (starches and sugars). Carbohydrates are great foods *but* they are horribly addictive and cause metabolic syndrome (also known as 'insulin resistance' and 'pre-diabetes' – see below). In the past, metabolic syndrome was an essential tool to allow primitive man to survive the winter: when the autumn windfall came, the carbohydrate craving was switched on as our forebears feasted on the natural and delicious harvests of grains, root vegetables, pulses and fruit. This made them fat (food storage and winter insulation) and lethargic (energy conservation) – ideal for getting through winter on a restricted diet.

Most of the time, we should be fuelling our body with a few sugars (from carbo-hydrates and proteins) and lots of short chain fatty acids (from fat and fibre). If sugar is available, our body always uses this first – this is because we can only store small amounts of this fuel as glycogen. Fat is so important because we can store vast amounts of this fuel (as fat) for winter survival. Evolution does not like us dipping into precious survival foods without good reason.

Fuelling our body with excess carbohydrate leads to the forerunner of diabetes – namely, metabolic syndrome (characterised by high carbohydrate 'junk food' diets, leading to obesity, high blood pressure, arterial damage and degenerative disease). With time, metabolic syndrome disables and kills. Years of carbohydrate-based diets and metabolic syndrome dump us prematurely on the evolutionary scrap heap.

Carbohydrates and disease

A high-carbohydrate diet overwhelms the ability of the liver to deal with it and this switches on the hormonal response which inhibits the burning of fat as fuel – this hormonal response is primarily the release of insulin (insulin lays down fat) but also mild hypothyroidism can result. Of course, in our evolutionary past, when the autumn feast of ripe fruit etc came to an end, because it ran out or rotted, 'primitive' Homo sapiens switched back into the normal fat-burning mode that we call ketosis.

On the other hand, we modern Western humans live in a state of permanent autumn because we can; the 'autumn feast' is permanently available in our supermarkets. We power our bodies with addictive high-carbohydrate foods that are constantly, conveniently and cheaply available. We are in constant metabolic syndrome with all the short-term (fat and fatigue) and long-term (heart disease, cancer and dementia) problems associated with that (see our book *Prevent and Cure Diabetes* for more details).

> *To every thing there is a season...*
>
> Ecclesiastes 3, King James V version, *The Bible*

High-carbohydrate diets mean that our glycogen sponge – which I will explain next – is constantly saturated. And therein lies the rub. It is not sugar per se that is the problem; it is too much sugar. How come?

The glycogen sponge

On eating, foods are digested and absorbed so there is a tsunami of products of digestion pouring into the portal vein, the blood drainage system from the gut that goes straight to the liver. The contents of the portal vein include a mixed soup of goodies and baddies. The liver does an amazing job to detoxify the baddies and store the goodies. Indeed, if this toxic soup bypassed the liver, we would rapidly fall into dementia and unconsciousness. This is precisely what happens in liver failure.

All carbohydrates are absorbed as sugars and these are a mixed blessing – yes, they are a useful raw material for the synthesis of DNA, RNA, ATP (the energy molecule) and to detoxify via the process of glucuronidation. Some sugar can also be used as fuel. On the other hand, too much sugar spilling over into the systemic (whole-body) bloodstream is damaging; it is sticky stuff and sticks to arteries (arteriosclerosis), feeds cancer cells, feeds infections and drives dementia and degenerative disease.

The primary control of blood sugar is carried out by the 'glycogen sponge' of the liver and muscle cells. Think of these as pantries where sugar can be temporarily stored as it floods in after a meal, then is slowly released according to demand. Returning to the analogy of a tsunami, engineers use their own form of a glycogen sponge for when flooding occurs. They build diversion canals to move water away from areas where it is accumulating and then store such 'excess' water in temporary holding ponds, thus averting damage to life, limb and property.

No problem at all, but if we overwhelm our glycogen-sponge pantry, if the holding ponds cannot accommodate the sugar tsunami, then the sugar will spill into the bloodstream and that triggers a host of hormonal responses which we call metabolic syndrome. In our analogy, the temporary holding ponds become full and so flood, thus causing the very damage they were intended to avert.

The key to consuming carbs is to make sure we never overwhelm our glycogen sponges. We can do that simply by measuring ketones (see Chapter 4).

The fermenting upper gut

The human gut is almost unique in the mammal world. The upper gut (oesophagus, stomach and small intestine) is a sterile carnivorous gut (like a dog's) designed for digesting protein and fat. The lower gut is a fermenting vegetarian gut designed to utilise fibre (like a horse, except humans cannot ferment that very tough fibre, cellulose). This allows humans to deal with many different foods and in part explains our success as a species. This system works perfectly until we overwhelm our ability to deal with sugars and starches. Bacteria and yeasts can then colonise the hitherto sterile upper gut and start fermenting. This creates nasty symptoms and pathology. Why?

1. Foods are fermented to toxins such as ethyl, propyl and butyl alcohols, D lactate, ammonia compounds, hydrogen, hydrogen sulphide and much else. This fermentation is otherwise known as the 'auto-brewery syndrome'. All these nasties have the potential to poison us, and this includes causing foggy brain. I just need a glass of wine to appreciate that fact!
2. Colonies of microbes – bacteria and fungi – build up and are then further colonised by viruses (so-called bacteriophages). Fermenting microbes produce bacterial endotoxins, fungal mycotoxins and viral particles.
3. These toxins spill over into the portal vein and so to the liver. The liver uses up much energy and raw materials to deal with these toxins. This is debilitating.
4. The gases generated by upper gut fermentation cause burping and bloating. They may distend the gut, and this is painful.
5. Microbes move into the lining of the gut and this low-grade inflammation results in a 'leaky gut'. This means that acid cannot be concentrated in the stomach because it leaks out as fast as it is secreted in. Acid is an essential part of digestion because:

a) it is necessary to start the digestion of protein
b) it is necessary for the absorption of minerals
c) it sterilises the upper gut and protects us from infections
d) it determines gut emptying: a non-acid stomach does not empty correctly and this drives reflux, oesophagitis, heartburn and hiatus hernia.

6. Microbes, dead and alive, and undigested foods leak into the bloodstream and drive pathology at distant sites. This is a major cause of pathology, including inflammatory bowel disease, arthritis, fibromyalgia, connective tissue disease, autoimmunity, interstitial cystitis, urticaria, venous ulcers, intrinsic asthma, kidney disease, possibly psychosis, and other brain pathologies such as Parkinson's disease.

7. Chronic inflammation of the lining of the gut results in cancer, especially of the stomach and oesophagus. Both are on the increase. Diet is the main reason, followed by acid-blocking drugs. These drugs also drive osteoporosis.

Fermentation of fibre by friendly microbes should take place in the colon, the lower gut/large intestine. The gases which result and make you fart are hydrogen and methane. These farts are odourless. Put a match to them and they will explode …not that I recommend this for diagnostic purposes! If your farts are offensive, then that is because you have overwhelmed your digestion upstream and proteins are being fermented in your colon – rotting meat stinks. Short gut transit time will have a similar effect. Professor Glenn Gibson, a food microbiologist from the University of Reading, divides people into 'inflammables' and 'smellies' – the inflammables (hydrogen and methane) have normal gut fermentation and the smellies (hydrogen sulphide) do not.[2] This is a risk factor for bowel cancer among many other problems that we will look at next.

The common carbohydrate-driven medical problems

Accelerated ageing

Degeneration, diabetes and dementia, coronaries and cancer are all driven by carbohydrates. There is much more detail in our comprehensive book *Ecological Medicine* but we list the key problems here as essential to *why* we should all be eating a PK diet.

Accelerated immune suppression

There is no need to die in a pandemic… provided you are not overwhelming your body with sugars. Not only is the PK diet highly protective against the above diseases of Westerners, but it is also highly protective against infection. Throughout evolution, populations have been controlled by infectious disease, with cholera estimated to have killed a third of all humans who ever existed and the Black Death responsible for killing a third of the population of Europe during the 14th Century.‡ With our modern CV19 pandemic, death rates are more than doubled in those with diabetes and tripled in the obese. We know there will be other pandemics to come which may well be more lethal than the current one. Those people clever enough to work out that the PK diet is the one we should be doing *and* who are disciplined enough to hold it in place will be the survivors of this plague. Natural selection and the survival of the fittest will prevail. Perhaps this provides you with the extra incentive to act now!

Why paleo? No dairy

Many passages and quotations from bygone days extol the virtues of dairy products, especially milk. *Exodus* 33.3 talks of the 'land flowing with milk and honey' as a promised land. Lady Macbeth fears that her husband is too full of the 'milk of human kindness', again placing 'milk' as a positive notion in our psyche. So, the belief that dairy products are healthy for us is very entrenched in our culture. It is well then to pause and consider this 'received wisdom' and the actual facts.

> *We do not receive wisdom; we must discover it for ourselves.*
> Marcel Proust, 10 July 1871 – 18 November 1922, French novelist,
> critic and essayist.

‡ **Historical aside:** It is conjectured that one reason why some church steeples are crooked is because during the Black Death so many skilled stonemasons died that this meant unskilled labourers had to finish off the job. Sometimes these labourers used unseasoned wood, which can cause some twisting until after about 50 years, when the wood is fully seasoned, and this can cause curving of the steeple. Often too much lead was laid down on the roof, and this can result in uneven forces causing twisting in the steeple, and also had the unintended consequence of much theft of church property centuries later. Also, it is thought that some unskilled labourers laid down too much stone, thinking this would strengthen the steeple, when in fact it set up force systems that buckled the entire structure. Some steeples fell down as a result of these mistakes, but some survived in their crooked form. So, the next time you see a crooked steeple on a 14th Century church, think Black Death.

However, before we do this, let us not forget Cleopatra, who had other uses for milk. It is often quoted, with much historical evidence, that Cleopatra bathed in sour donkey's milk to improve the look of her skin. The logic goes that when milk sours, lactose is converted by bacteria into lactic acid and this in turn causes the surface layer of the skin to peel off, leaving new, smoother, blemish-free skin underneath. Indeed, lactic acid is an example of an alpha hydroxy acid and such acids are used in modern-day cosmetics for 'wrinkle-free skin', so this story is plausible. However, this is an early example of symptom suppression – I prefer more natural and sustainable methods for obtaining healthy skin – please see our book *Ecological Medicine*.

There is also a less well recognised purpose for which Cleopatra utilised milk; the great Queen is remembered as what we may call a toxicologist these days – she first started administering her poisons in wine but when that method became too well known and suspected, she turned to milk as her preferred medium of delivery. Cleopatra was very methodical. She conducted many experiments and tested different poisons to see their effects, lethality and dosage that would be needed to cause death, along with the amount of suffering caused by the various toxins. These experiments were carried out on men (her chosen target!) and often Marc Antony was forced to witness them, perhaps as a warning? So, with that in mind, let us return to why it is that dairy products, even when not mixed with Cleopatra's poisons, are so dangerous to us.

Why dairy products are so dangerous to health

Dairy products from the cow, goat and sheep have created numerous health problems in Westerners because: they are major allergens for many; they cause food intolerance in many others; they contain growth promoters that are a risk for cancer in everybody; and they are also a risk factor for autoimmunity, heart disease and osteoporosis in us all. Read on.

Dairy products are major allergens

Dairy products cause allergy reactions in, I estimate, at least 20% of the UK population. Charles Darwin suffered ill-health for 40 years but was cured when he stopped consuming dairy products. The allergen (milk protein – casein) remains the same throughout life but the target organ changes. Newborn babies may suffer projectile vomiting due to the pyloric stenosis triggered by milk protein. Even if Mum is breastfeeding, this tough protein will get into her breastmilk if she is consuming it. Three-month colic is typical of dairy allergy. However, the target organ then changes – next we see toddler diarrhoea. The tot may grow out of this problem but then becomes catarrhal, with snotty nose, snoring, cough and recurrent upper respiratory tract infections, including otitis media, tonsillitis, sinusitis and bronchitis. Asthma may be diagnosed.

Later on in life, dairy allergy manifests with sleep apnoea, migraine, irritable bowel syndrome, depression and arthritis. I get a painful hip if I eat dairy products; as a child I was told I had 'growing pains' – what a joke! Indeed, I used to chat away with the late Dr Honor Anthony, Consultant Allergist. She maintained that nearly all cases of arthritis were caused by allergy. At the time I dismissed this notion; I now know she was absolutely spot on!

If arthritis is not from allergy to foods, then it probably results from allergy to microbes spilling over into the bloodstream from the fermenting gut. This is called 'bacterial translocation'.[2, 3]

The link between forms of arthritis and microbes is also well documented.[4, 5]

In the long term, chronic undiagnosed allergy often results in fatigue. I see many patients with chronic fatigue syndrome and myalgic encephalitis (CFS/ME). A particularly common progression is the undiagnosed dairy-allergic child picking up recurrent infections, especially tonsillitis, then getting glandular fever and switching into a post-viral chronic fatigue syndrome. (See our book *Diagnosis and Treatment of Chronic Fatigue Syndrome and Myalgic Encephalitis – it's mitochondria not hypochondria*).

Dairy products cause lactose intolerance

Lactose intolerance results when one lacks the enzyme to digest milk sugar (lactose). It occurs in 5% of Northern Europeans and 90% of Africans and Asians. If lactose cannot be digested, it gets fermented in the gut by microbes to produce some, or all, of the symptoms of upper fermenting gut, such as bloating, pain, reflux, nausea, indigestion and diarrhoea (again, see our book *Ecological Medicine*). Many cultures, such as those in the Near and Far East, do not traditionally drink fresh milk or use cream for this reason. They can only eat fermented milks or ghee.[§]

[§] Footnote: For those who are interested in learning more about this topic, there is an interesting website, complete with links to studies, entitled 'Lactose Intolerance by Ethnicity and Region'.[6]

Dairy products are growth promoters

Milk has evolved over millions of years as the perfect nutrition for the mammalian baby. Mammalian babies need to grow and become fit and strong very quickly so that they can escape predators. This would be especially true of the ancestors of our modern cows, goats and sheep. Once born there was little their mothers could do to protect them from predators. Within a few hours of birth, they had to keep up with the herd. Milk was and still is full of growth promoters. Those calves, kids and lambs grew very quickly.

Human children fed dairy products also grow quickly. It is entirely natural that they suckle human breast milk but entirely unnatural that they consume the milk of other mammals. When challenged by the question, 'Are dairy products not natural foods', longstanding advocate of paleo diets, Dr Lorain Cordain, replied: 'Have you ever tried milking a wild bison?'

We now have a generation of youngsters who are taller and fatter than ever before, partly because they are consuming dairy products. Carbohydrates in the form of sugar and refined starches further have their effect on height and weight. Being tall and fat are both known risk factors for getting cancer. Indeed, the first positive nutritional step for preventing and treating cancer is to cut out all dairy products, sugars and carbohydrates. The Million Women Study concluded that: 'Cancer incidence increases with increasing adult height for most cancer sites. The relation between height and total cancer RR [relative risk] is similar in different populations.'[7]

We all produce about 10,000 DNA mutations every second. Some will be early cancers. The immune system is well able to identify these rogue cells and kill them off before they cause problems, but, if they grow too quickly, driven by dairy products and carbohydrates, they overwhelm the immune system's ability to cope with them and so tumours develop. As we age the imperative to avoid all dairy products increases.

Dairy products increase the risk of autoimmunity

We are seeing epidemics of autoimmunity, with one in 20 of the population currently affected. Of particular concern is the rise in type 1 diabetes in children. The three known major risk factors for this are vaccination, vitamin D deficiency and consumption of dairy products. The mechanism of this is probably due to circulating antibodies against cow's milk protein which then cross-react with the self – in the case of type 1 diabetes, with the Islets of Langerhan in the pancreas which are our insulin factories. There are numerous studies linking the consumption of dairy products with type 1 diabetes. One by Gerstein

(1994), concluded that: 'Early cow's milk exposure may be an important determinant of subsequent type 1 diabetes and may increase the risk approximately 1.5 times.'[8]

A Finnish study of 690 type 1 diabetic children was more direct in its conclusion: 'This is the first observational study to show that early introduction of dairy products is independently associated with an increased risk of IDDM. Adjustment for mother's education and age, child's birth order, or birth weight did not affect the results.'[9]

Dairy products increase the risk of osteoporosis

When I suggest people stop consuming dairy the immediate riposte is, 'What about my calcium?' and 'Will I not get osteoporosis?'. In fact, calcium is a side issue. There is plenty of calcium (and more important than calcium is magnesium) in PK foods. However, two greater issues are: (1) How well is calcium (and magnesium) absorbed? And (2) Where is it deposited?

Vitamin D is the key. Vitamin D greatly enhances the absorption of calcium (and magnesium) but, as importantly, stimulates its deposition in bone. We should all take at least 5000 iu of vitamin D daily.

Indeed, magnesium is more important than calcium in the prevention and treatment of osteoporosis. The proportion of calcium to magnesium in dairy products is 10:1 but our physiological requirements are 2:1. Since calcium and magnesium compete for absorption, dairy products induce a magnesium deficiency. It may be that this is part of the mechanism by which dairy products increase the risk of osteoporosis.[10]

Dairy products are a risk factor for heart disease

A good friend and colleague, Dr David Freed, produced a paper called 'The Cow and the Coronary'. It concluded that the non-fat aspects of milk strongly correlated with deaths from heart disease. Milk factor antibodies bind to platelets, resulting in sticky blood: 'We suggest that non-fat aspects of milk, particularly the Ca/Mg ratio, lactose and MFGM antigens, have specific coronary atherogenic effects, both biochemical and immunological, and the simultaneous attack from these three directions may explain why this foodstuff has such a strong effect.'[11]

Conclusion

Given all the risks above, the conclusion must be not to eat dairy products. However, butter may be okay. If you suffer no symptoms or diseases and are otherwise completely well, then I do permit just this one dairy product. Dairy fat is the safest part of dairy products. Better than butter is ghee as it is pure fat –to make it, butter has been warmed so the dangerous cow's milk protein has floated to the top and has been scraped off as a white scum leaving clear yellow pure fat behind.

Why paleo? No gluten grains

Cooks and gourmets love gluten because its stickiness allows them to make breads and biscuits, cakes and cookies, pastries, pastas and pies, but this adhesive is also toxic. Gluten is a major allergen and risk factor for autoimmunity. I know of two patients whose autoimmune thyrotoxicosis is clearly triggered by gluten.

Worse, many grains contain toxic lectins. Lectins are 'plant antibiotics' – substances evolved to make that plant as toxic as possible to prevent it being eaten to death.

Another consideration is pesticide-related toxicity. Many modern grains are genetically modified, not for reasons of good nutrition but so that they are more tolerant of pesticides. In consequence, these grains carry a high pesticide burden. One of the most toxic is glyphosate which chemically is an organophosphate (OP). OPs are known carcinogens and mutagens (drive cell mutation) and also inhibit our energy-producing mitochondria; this explains the severe fatigue of 'sheep dip flu', Gulf War syndrome and aerotoxic syndrome (see our book *Diagnosis and Treatment of Chronic Faitgue Syndrome and Myalgic Encephalitis*). Glyphosate is particularly toxic to the kidneys.

At a recent conference I attended, the consensus was that gluten grains and corn are unsafe for human consumption and should be reserved for animal feed only. Poor animals. And poor us when we eat those animals.

The starting point to prevent all disease

The PK diet is the starting point to prevent all disease, from cancer and coronaries to chronic fatigue and Covid19.

Chapter 1

I had to work in the field of ecological medicine for four decades, see over 20,000 patients and write several books with Craig, to convince myself that paleo-ketogenic was the diet we should all be eating. Since I do not ask my patients to do anything that I do not do myself, I started this diet and I have to say that this was with a with a great sense of bereavement. Was I going to miss all those foods I loved and had become used to eating? However, having established myself on this diet I now know that this is what I shall be eating for the rest of my life.

As I get older, and perhaps wiser, I find myself spending more and more time discussing diet. This is the starting point for treating absolutely everything. However, it is also the most difficult thing I ask my patients to do. If I give my patients a list of interventions they need to make, they tend to cherry-pick, choosing the easy things first. This has usually meant that diet is the last thing to be tackled.

Diet is the *first* thing we could and should be doing to restore health. The upside of this is that diet is something we can all do – the treatment is in your shopping baskets and kitchens. You don't need any physicians, pills or potions. Dietary changes are empowering – they allow us to take back control of our health. However, dietary changes are also the most difficult for all the reasons that we detail in our earlier book, *Prevent and Cure Diabetes*: addiction, habit and convenience.[¶] The job of this current book is to try to make these dietary changes much easier.

My job is to get patients well as quickly as possible. I used to try to be nice and pussy-foot about, trying dairy-free diets, gluten-free diets, low-carbohydrate diets or whatever. These days I am much nastier as I cruelly say 'My job is to get you well, not to entertain you'. I now start off with the toughest diet in order to get my patients well as quickly as possible. Once recovered, they can then, as I call it, 'do a deal with the devil'. Of course, one can get away with some foods on the occasional treat basis so long as one is consciously aware of what one is doing and is determined to get back on the wagon straight after.

[¶] **Note from Craig:** Before becoming a ketogenic, I would eat at least six packets of ready-salted crisps a day. I even had a stash *and* a secret stash, in case of emergencies, just like Hugh Laurie's *Gregory House* and his Vicodin (in the TV series *House*). I stopped all crisps on one day and have never gone back. It is not easy though – even the rustle of a crisp packet brings back memories and I have a Pavlovian response of salivation (see page 126) to this day.

> *Sometimes, you must be cruel to be kind*
>
> Old English Proverb

Having said all that, it has never been easier to go PK. We now have fabulous PK replacements for bread, biscuits, cakes and puddings. The dairy alternatives are superb. You may feel initially deprived when you can no longer give in to your carbohydrate addiction but that is the same for all addicts whether smokers, vapers, drinkers, gamblers or jabbers. You will rediscover your true health, energy and taste buds.

> *Before you heal someone, ask him if he's willing to give up the things that make him sick.*
>
> Hippocrates

Just do it!

Chapter 2

What is the PK diet?

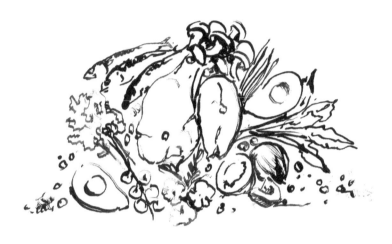

The PK diet is paleo (no gluten grains or dairy products except perhaps for butter and ghee – see Chapter 1 and below), ketogenic (low-carbohydrate: no sugar, fruit sugar, grains, pulses and root vegetables), high-fat and high-fibre. It is *not* a high-protein diet. Modern PK demands extra micronutrients. One can eat some carbohydrates, but too much (read on) and the diet fails. The aim is to fuel the body primarily with fat and fibre, occasionally with starches and sugars. Paleo *plus* ketogenic is better than either on its own.

> 'The combination is more than the sum of its pieces'
> 'The whole is greater than the sum of its parts.'
>
> Aristotle, 384 – 322 BC

Low carbohydrate

We all want simple answers to a simple question – which carbohydrates can I eat and which not? Actually, you can eat any carbohydrate depending on the amount and how addicted you are.

Addiction

I am a sugar addict. Give me one biscuit and I will be craving more – the rest of the packet is not safe. I have the discipline to say no to the first biscuit but not to the second. I can get away with 85% chocolate – my appetite is satisfied with two squares – so that tells me I am not an addict for this food.

Take great care with sugars. Many modern fruit varieties are so sweet that they too switch on addictive eating. As with all addictions, you must just say 'No!' Fruit-aholics have a further problem because the fruit sugar fructose inhibits glycogen phosphorylase – this is the enzyme which allows the glycogen sponge (page 5) to be squeezed dry. Fruit-aholics therefore suffer from hypoglycaemia (low blood sugar) because they can't 'correct' the situation (bring the blood sugar level back up), even with glycogen. This explains why corn-syrup, so beloved by Americans, is such a pernicious sweetener as the main sugar within it is fructose.

Even non-sugar sweeteners, be they natural (sorbitol, stevia, erythritol) or artificial (aspartame, saccharine, sucralose) switch on that terrible physical and psychological craving. It is best to avoid these completely. Importantly, avoiding sweeteners will change your taste buds and what was once craved becomes sickly. The PK gourmet *occasionally* uses sweeteners modestly as flavour enhancers but do not over-do this.

Sugar is as addictive as alcohol!

> *First you take a drink, then the drink takes a drink, then the drink takes you.*
> F. Scott Fitzgerald, 1896 – 1940, *The Great Gatsby*

Amount

Many feel they have to eat a certain volume of food to 'fill up' and feel 'satisfied'. However, much of that 'satisfaction' derives from a hitherto unrecognised addictive carbohydrate hit. Eat slowly, chewing every mouthful, as chewing satisfies. Use foods that are tough or high-fibre and require much chewing (raw vegetables, salads and coleslaws) and which cannot be gobbled.

What to eat

A reasonable starting point for most is the division set out below into: foods that are 0% carbs (you can eat any amount); foods that are less than 5% carbs; foods that are 5-10% carbs (care needed); and foods that are 10% or more carbs (avoid completely). Also see Appendix 1 which gives the carbohydrate content of commonly consumed foods.

Zero carbs

You can eat as much as you like of:
- Fats (solid at room temperature) – saturated fats for energy, such as lard, butter (ideally ghee, so long as you are sure you are not allergic to dairy; I am … dammit), goose fat, coconut oil, palm oil. These are also ideal for cooking as they can withstand high temperatures.
- Oils (liquid at room temperature) – unsaturated fats are fuels too but also contain essential omega 3 and 6 and also omega 9 fatty acids. Hemp oil is ideal, containing the perfect proportion of omega 6 to omega 3 – that is, 4:1. These must be cold pressed and not used for cooking or you risk 'flipping' them into toxic trans fats (see Chapter 3).
- Fibre – this is often included in the carb count of foods and leads to some confusion so it is important to understand what food labelling means.

A note on food labelling

When 'counting carbs', we are looking for what we call the 'net carbs figure'. This is the carb content *minus* fibre (fibre is carbohydrate that can't be digested by humans) or, to put it another way, 'net carbs' is starches plus sugars.

Labelling differs between the US and EU (including the UK) – when reading food labels, one must understand the differences in what is disclosed. For example, if an item, in America, contains 5 grams of what is called 'total carbohydrates', out of which 2 grams consist of what is called 'dietary fibre', then the 'net carbs' content of this product is 3 grams (5 minus 2). In other words, the label will disclose 'total carbohydrates' of 5 grams and within that figure **sub-disclose** 2 grams of fibre.

In the UK, and the EU, net carbs are already calculated within nutritional labels. Simple/complex carbohydrates (sugars/starches) are disclosed as one entity ('carbohydrate') and dietary fibre is separately labelled as 'fibre'. Hence there is no need to calculate 'net carbs' content for a product that follows EU labelling rules – just use the 'carbohydrate' disclosed figure. So, to go back to the US example above, disclosure in the UK/EU would be 'Carbohydrate 3 grams' and 'Fibre 2 grams'.

However, in all cases, please do check the labels as some companies use different methods even to those noted above.

Less than 5% carbs

The most important foods that have less than 5% carb are listed below. See Appendix 1 (page 195) for more. These can be eaten freely:

- **linseed**. See Chapter 8 for PK bread and Chapter 10 for PK porridge and muesli. Linseed is 27% fibre and 2% carb.
- **coconut cream**. I love Grace coconut milk which has a 2% carb content; it pours like cream and is a great dairy alternative.
- **Brazil** and **pecan nuts** are less than 5% carb.
- **salad** (lettuce, cucumber, tomato, pepper etc) plus avocado pears and olives (phew! I love them both).
- **green leafy vegetables**.
- **mushrooms and fungi**. A difficulty with this diet is eating enough fat; these foods are great for frying as they mop up delicious, saturated fats.
- **fermented foods** (sauerkraut, kefir) as the carb content has been fermented out by microbes.

Then, though the following are not high-carb, take care with:
- meat, fish, shellfish and eggs – don't have too much as excessive amounts of protein can be converted back to carbohydrate, in a process called gluconeogenesis. See Chapter 3 (page 34) to calculate your protein needs.
- coffee and tea – drink these in moderation only as they are addictive and may switch on carbohydrate craving.

Between 5% and 10% carbs

Take care with foods that are 5-10% carb. These include:
*   berries
*   some nuts – e.g. almonds
*   herbs and spices – these do have a carb content but in the small amounts normally
    used these are not going to spike sugar levels.

Over 10% carbs

Take great care with all foods that are more than 10% carb as they switch on addictive
eating. I know – as I have said, I too am an addict. These include:
*   all grains
*   all pulses
*   fruits (apart from berries) and their juices
*   many nuts and seeds
*   'junk' foods, which are characterised by a high-carb content and addictive potential,
    including crisps (sorry, Craig).

Micronutrient supplements

Why supplements are needed

You need to take micronutrient supplements for life to compensate for the deficiencies
resulting from contemporary farming and food production methods. Primitive humans
did not require nutritional supplements, but modern Western humans, even those eating a
PK diet, do for the following obvious and logical reasons:
*   There is now a one-way movement of minerals from the soil to plants, animals and
    humans. We no longer recycle these minerals back to the land and therefore there is
    a net depletion of minerals from the soil and ultimately from food. This is especially
    true of vitamin B12 – lack of optimal levels in humans is very common. (Whilst
    vitamin B12 can be synthesised in the human gut, this occurs in the colon whence
    it cannot be absorbed. Humans have to eat meat, fish or eggs to get vitamin B12.
    Vegans are invariably deficient and must supplement; vegetarians often are.)

- Moreover, if plants do not contain minerals, they then cannot make the vitamins and essential fatty acids that are vital for animal and human life.
- Most of our crops, including those which are used to feed farm animals, are annual crops, so that only the upper few inches of soil are exploited. This nutritious topsoil is being rapidly depleted by modern farming techniques.
- The mineral deficiencies which result increase the need for pesticides and herbicides. These toxic chemicals create further problems downstream because:
  o Many pesticides, such as glyphosate, work by chelating minerals in soil, thereby reducing mineral availability to plants,… and so further increasing the need for pesticides!
  o The use of nitrogen fertilisers and pesticides reduces the humus content (the mycorrhiza – a symbiotic association composed of fungus and the roots of vascular plants) of soil and therefore plants will malabsorb minerals,… and so further increase the need for pesticides.
  o Pesticides increase the toxic load in food; this toxic load requires more micronutrients for the body to detoxify and excrete them.
- Genetically modified crops – genetic modification is largely done to develop pesticide-resistant strains rather than for improving micronutrient density; more pesticide is therefore used, exacerbating the above problems.
- Crops may be bred or genetically modified for their appearance or keeping qualities, at the expense of good micronutrient content.
- Crops may be bred or genetically modified for high sugar content to appeal to our sweet-craving palates. Primitive man's idea of an autumn treat was a crab apple.*
- Modern man does not exercise as much as primitive man and therefore needs less food; less food means fewer micronutrients. Even recently, actual calorie consumption has fallen – in Britain, we eat 600 fewer calories daily than 30 years ago.[1]
- Refined carbohydrates require more micronutrients to deal with them than are present within them; these foods deplete nutrients indirectly.

---

* **Note from Craig:** This is definitely true of raspberries – I have to hunt high and low to find the tart raspberries that I love. When I visit, Sarah often gives me a bag of her raspberries, tart as you like (the raspberries, not Sarah!).

For further reading please see the Nutrition Security Institute's White Paper: *Human Health, the Nutritional Quality of Harvested Food and Sustainable Farming Systems*[2] which stated back in 1936 that: 'The alarming fact is that foods – fruits, vegetables and grains – now being raised on millions of acres of land that no longer contains enough of certain needed nutrients, are starving us - no matter how much we eat of them.'

By contrast with all other animals, humans, fruit bats and guineapigs cannot make their own vitamin C. We can consume sufficient to get us to child-bearing age, but this is not sufficient for optimal health and longevity. My dog Nancy eats a pure meat diet but does not get scurvy because she can make her own vitamin C. The 'recommended daily amount' (RDA) for vitamin C in humans is 30 milligrams; this may stop you getting scurvy[†], but it is far too low for optimal health. One report states a 70 kilo (155 lb) goat makes 13,000 milligrams (13 grams) of vitamin C daily. Linus Pauling, the only person to win two unshared Nobel prizes, advocated up to 14 grams daily (see *Ecological Medicine* for much more detail).

Sunshine deficiency and sunshine phobia plague those living away from the equator. Vitamin D deficiency is pandemic in Westerners. We all need at least one hour of full-body exposure to sunshine daily which provides about 10,000 iu of vitamin D for normal vitamin D blood levels. There is, however, a further problem. 'Normal' levels in the blood are set too low so many people are told they have enough vitamin D to prevent rickets or osteomalacia, but this is insufficient for optimum health.

As often is the case and we have seen in relation to vitamin C, recommended daily allowances (RDAs) are set to avoid certain illnesses, rather than to optimise health.

Finally, our need for salt increases with a PK diet because of improvements in our metabolism. Yes, salt is an essential – see Chapter 16.

[†] **Note on scurvy:** Some Americans still refer to us Brits as 'Limeys'. This slang term derives from the 19th Century practice of the Royal Navy of adding lemon juice to the daily ration of grog (watered-down rum) as a means of supplying just about enough vitamin C to prevent scurvy. At that time, the words 'lemon' and 'lime' were used interchangeably to refer to citrus fruits and so Limey was used to describe, first, Royal Navy sailors, and then later, all Brits. Those interested in slang terms for the British may like the *New York Times* article 'On Language; Brits, Tommies, Poms, Limeys and Kippers'[3]

What supplements are needed?

To compensate for the above problems, to maintain your health, take daily:
- A good multivitamin.
- Sunshine salt: 5 grams/one teaspoonful daily sprinkled on food (see below) and/or used in cooking (see Chapter 17).
- Vitamin C: 5 grams as ascorbic acid dissolved in 2 litres of water and drunk little and often through the day.

Adjust the dose with age, disease and chronic inflammation, as follows:
- A good multivitamin.
- Sunshine salt as above.
- Vitamin D 10,000 iu daily (this is perfectly safe in addition to the vitamin D in Sunshine salt so long as you avoid excessive calcium as in dairy products) [what happens with excessive calcium? What is excessive calcium? If someone is drinking lots of mineral – usually high in calcium – could that be too much?]
- Essential fatty acids, such as hemp oil 1 dessertspoon daily, possibly with extra omega 6 and 3 (evening primrose oil and fish oils) in the proportion 4:1.
- Vitamin C: 5-15 grams (yes, I mean 5000 to 15,000 milligrams, and no that is not a big dose) daily. See our books *Ecological Medicine* and *The Infection Game* for more detail on vitamin C and using it to 'bowel tolerance'.

What the PK diet is not

The PK diet is *not* a high-protein diet, nor is it the Paleo diet (too high in carbs) or a Ketogenic diet (high in dairy products), but a fusion of the best aspects of the two. Table 2.1 gives a summary of the pros and cons of eight commonly followed different diet types.

Table 2.1: The pros and cons of eight common diets

Diet	Pros	Cons	Notes: See our book *Prevent and Cure Diabetes* for details of all the below
Normal 'Western' diet	Westerners no longer suffer from starvation, but this diet has little else to commend it	High in refined carbohydrates such as sugar, fruit and fruit juice, potato, cereal grains and 'junk food'	Induces metabolic syndrome with all its complications, including fatigue, obesity, diabetes, tooth decay, arterial and heart disease, cancer and dementia
		Low in fat	'Fat is the most valuable food known to Man' to quote Dr John Yudkin, founding Professor, Department of Dietetics, Queen Elizabeth College, London. Increased risk of dementia ('type 3 diabetes')
		Low in fibre	Increased risk of gut cancers
		Low in protein	We have to eat more to satisfy our protein appetite, so we eat more calories and get fat
		Low in micro-nutrients	Accelerated ageing
		No 'real' fermented foods	The consumption of live ferments extends longevity
		Alcohol	Highly toxic and addictive
		High in the major allergens – namely gluten and dairy	Food allergy and intolerance are estimated to cause ill health in over one third of Westerners (see our book *Ecological Medicine*)
	Easy, convenient, cheap, quick...	...but addictive and toxic	I believe that sugar and refined carbohy-drates are more dangerous to health than smoking; they are more addictive because they are still socially acceptable

Diet	Pros	Cons	Notes: See our book *Prevent and Cure Diabetes* for details of all the below
Paleo diet	No gluten grains No dairy No refined sugar Includes fermented foods		Avoids the major allergens that commonly cause irritable bowel syndrome, psychiatric conditions, migraine and headaches, asthma, eczema, arthritis and many other such inflammatory conditions (see our book *Ecological Medicine*)
		Allows fruit, potatoes, non-gluten cereals and natural sugars; may be high in sugar and starch	This can induce metabolic syndrome
Ketogenic diet such as Atkins	High in fat Low in carbs High in micro-nutrients		Highly effective for reversing obesity and diabetes because the protein appetite is satisfied and the ketosis which ensues means you literally exhale and pee out calories
		High in dairy products	These are a common cause of allergy, growth promotion (so increased risk of cancer), and a major risk factor for heart disease and osteoporosis
		High in artificial sweeteners	Many, such as aspartame, are toxic, triggering headaches, depression, seizures, attention-deficit disorder (ADD) as well as cancer and birth defects. Sweeteners maintain the sweet-taste addiction
Low-fat slimming diets	I can think of no pros for this awful diet	Often rely on carbs as a fuel source	The body ends up in the 'metabolic hinter-land' (see Chapter 5) unable to get fuel from carbs or fat. This diet results in fatigue, foggy brain and feeling cold and depressed, which is why it is unsustainable. It requires massive determi-nation (which I, for one, do not possess). It does not switch off carbohydrate craving, does not permit fat burning except through starvation, and in the long term this results in yo-yo weight swings

		Low in fat	See page 25
		High in artificial sweeteners	See opposite
GAPS diet	A good step towards a PK diet…	…but allows fruit and cheese	For some this diet will be sufficient to solve their health problems, but fruit is a bag of sugar and as potentially dangerous as the white stuff. Dairy products are common allergens
Vegetarian	High in fibre	May be low in protein	Protein is essential for tissue healing and repair and our bodies know if we do have enough. Low-protein diets can therefore cause cravings and result in weight gain – this is called 'protein leverage'
		High in carbohy-drates	This can induce metabolic syndrome – see above
		High in allergens such as dairy and gluten	Not a good diet for the allergic – at least one third of the UK population suffer symptoms due to food allergy or intolerance
		May be low in micronutrients such as iron and vitamin B12	
Vegan	See above for Vegetarian plus dairy-free	See above for vegetarian	Ditto above for vegetarian
		Difficult to eat sufficient fat	Saturated fat is an essential fuel. Unsaturated fats are a vital raw material
		Often very low in protein	Again, protein leverage results in weight gain
		No vitamin B12 without supple-menting	Primitive man was an omnivore

Diet	Pros	Cons	Notes: See our book *Prevent and Cure Diabetes* for details of all the below
Many allergy exclusion diets	Low in allergens	May be high in carbohydrates. Can become too restricted and calorie-deficient	
The PK diet	High-fat High-fibre Low-carb Low-allergen Rich in micronutri-ents Low chemical and toxic burden Not addictive		The starting point for preventing and treating most diseases – but not all… Unfortunately it does not stop me falling off my horse; it just increases the desire to ride more
		Initial difficulties to keto-adapt, with a difficult passage through the metabolic hinterland Perceived as anti-social (because few others have woken up to the benefits)	Get organised and change the habits of a lifetime. All these 'cons' are solved by turning the pages of this book… read on, my friend!

Our bodies are our gardens, to the which our wills are gardeners.
Othello Act 1 Scene 3, William Shakespeare (April 1564 - 23 April 1616)

I must make one final point, just to expand on the perceived anti-social nature of the PK diet. You can eat this diet when you go out to a restaurant, but you will have to ask the waiter to leave out certain foods and add others in their place. Craig has found that this has often led to interesting discussions about why he is eating this way – a great way to educate people. 'Going against' the received wisdom is often difficult, but this journey is worth it and, remember that, as Voltaire (1694 – 1778) said, 'It is dangerous to be right in matters on which the established authorities are wrong.' The 'danger' here is social opprobrium.

Also, Walter de la Mare (1873 – 1956) said of (conventional) thoughts: 'It was a pity thoughts always ran the easiest way, like water in old ditches.'

So, again, we repeat our mantra – *Just do it*!

Chapter 3

Balancing up the PK diet

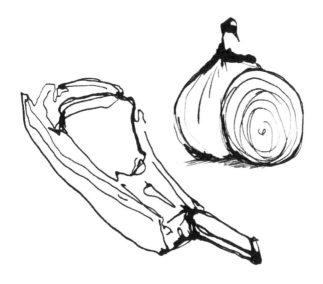

Calories: make sure you are eating enough

Many people chronically under-eat in a misguided attempt to keep their weight down.

However, under-eating puts the body into survival mode – it thinks there is a famine. The body and brain will cut down energy expenditure to deal with this abnormal state of affairs, resulting in physical fatigue, foggy brain and depression. You need enough food for energy (see our book The Energy Equation). Should you, however, wish to lose weight please turn to Chapter 24.

To calculate your calorie needs (also known as your basal metabolic rate (BMR)), use the Mifflin-St Jeor Equation as follows:

For men: BMR = 10 x weight in kg PLUS 6.25 x height in cm MINUS 5 x age in years PLUS 5

For women: BMR =10 x weight in kg PLUS 6.25 x height in cm MINUS 5 x age in years MINUS 161

Table 3.1 sets out how to do this calculation, including a worked example based on my weight, height and age.

If you do not fancy the maths, put your vital statistics into www.calculator.net/bmr-calculator.html and that will get your BMR just like that, but you will know now how it has been calculated.

Table 3.1: Calorie needs at rest (BMR) and when active

Steps **FIRST work out your BMR at rest**	Worked example **My vital statistics are: Weight 61 kg, height 168 cm, age 62**	Result for me
For women: BMR = 10 x weight (kg) PLUS 6.25 x height (cm) minus 5 x age (years) MINUS 161	10 x 61 kg = 610 PLUS 6.25 x 168 cm = 1050 MINUS 5 x 62 = 310 MINUS 161	610 PLUS 1050 MINUS 310 MINUS 161 My BMR is 1189 kcal
For men: BMR = 10 x weight (kg) PLUS 6.25 x height (cm) MINUS 5 x age (years) PLUS 5	Ditto above THEN ADD 5	If I were male, and Craig says I do have balls, the calculation would be: 610 PLUS 1050 MINUS 310 PLUS 5 My BMR would be 1355 kcal
THEN multiply your resting BMR by your activity factor to get your total energy expenditure: • Sedentary x 1.2 • Lightly active x 1.375 • Moderately active (moderate exercise 3-5 days) x 1.55 • Very active (hard exercise 6-7 days a week) x 1.725 • Super-active (hard exercise and sport and physical job) x 1.9	I am moderately active so I: MULTIPLY my BMR by a factor of 1.55 = 1189 x 1.55 = 1843	So my daily energy expenditure is 1843 kcal

Protein: not too little, not too much

Protein leverage: The body cannot store protein, but daily protein is essential for survival. We have a protein appetite which will make us crave food until that appetite has been satisfied. If you are eating a low-protein diet, you will be driven to eat more food. In that process you overeat carbs and fat and so expect to gain weight. Conversely, eat a high-protein diet and you tend to under-eat and lose weight. Get your protein intake right to help maintain a normal weight. (Note that a high-protein diet is not desirable as the body then has to deal with the toxic consequences of too much protein. Listen to your body and appetite – they will tell you how much you need.)

Table 3.2: How to calculate your protein requirement

Steps	Worked example – me	Result for me
FIRST work out your daily energy expenditure as above	My daily energy expenditure is 1843 kcal	
Then divide by 4 to give your daily protein need in grams (this need includes recycled protein from self)	DIVIDE 1843 by 4 = 461	
Then adjust for age protein requirements as % of daily energy requirement • Baby to adolescent: 15% • Young adult to 30 years: 18% • Pregnancy and breast-feeding: 20% • 30s: 17% • 40-60: 15% • 60-65: 18% • >65: 20%	I am 62 so I need my diet to be 18% protein 461 x 18/100 = 83	So, I need 83 grams of protein a day

Table 3.3: What and how much to eat to satisfy your protein requirement

Food	Protein content in grams (g) per 100 g	On the plate looks like... approx.	What I eat	My protein consumption approx
Eggs	13	Two eggs	Breakfast: 2 eggs	13
Beef	26	A medium beef burger		
Pork	31	Small pork chop	Supper, main course: pork chop	31
Bacon	Up to 39 depending on how fatty; 1 slice = 8 g			
Lamb	26	One lamb chop		
Chicken, duck	20	Whole breast or Whole leg		
Fish, fresh	29	A good chunk		
Prawns	25	A prawn 'cocktail' starter	Supper, starters: paté or fish	25
Brazil nuts	15		Snacks	10-15
				My total: 79-84

Once you have things roughly balanced out your body will do the rest. Appetite and desire for food are remarkably accurate once you have addiction out of the way. Interestingly, before I did this calculation what's listed in Table 3.3 was what I ate, so my brain and body had worked it out already.

Fibre: for the microbiome, fuel and more

Fibre is essential for the healthy gut and body. It is a carbohydrate, but not one that can be digested to sugar. This does lead to confusion with the carbohydrate count of foods because fibre is often included in the analysis. So, for example linseed is 29% carbohydrate of which 27% is fibre. We do not have the gut enzymes to digest fibre, but the lower gut (colon) contains kilograms of friendly bacteria which ferment it. This fermentation provides us with a fuel source of short chain fatty acids (yippee – more ketones!) and also essentials such as vitamin K, serotonin, several B vitamins and more that are synthesised in the process. The bulking effect of fibre shortens gut transit time to further reduce that toxic load (yes, turds are toxic). The friendly bacteria help to programme the immune system. Fibre protects us from many diseases.

Eat enough fibre until you are crapping like one of Denis Burkitt's Africans. Burkitt, a consultant surgeon, observed that indigenous Africans did not suffer Western diseases. For these Africans, normal defaecation meant twice daily squatting to produce a turd effortlessly (no straining), cucumber-size, no cracks, no balling, soft and inoffensive . To be precise, your number twos should become number 4s on the Bristol stool chart – and yes, you can purchase the T-shirt so emblazoned. (See the Bristol Stool Chart on WebMD at: www.webmd.com/digestive-disorders/poop-chart-bristol-stool-scale.) To achieve that which colorectal surgeons dream of you need to consume two to four PK buns (see Chapter 8: The PK bakery, page 81) or its fibre equivalent. Then invest in a squatty potty to produce the optimum angle of descent for evacuation; I was delighted to read that some have 'motion sensitive lights'.

As John Cummings and Amanda Engineer state in their 2017 article in Nutrition Research Review,[1] *Burkitt built on work by Peter Cleave and colleagues (physicians), Neil Painter (a surgeon) and Alec Walker (a biochemist) and went on to postulate that low-fibre diets led to heightened risks of becoming obese and developing coronary artery disease, diabetes and various large bowel diseases such as cancer and diverticulosis. Finding a common cause for such a wide variety of diseases was revolutionary. As a result, Burkitt was dubbed 'Fibre Man'.*

Fats and oils: essential fuels, building materials and hormone precursors

Fat is the most valuable food known to Man.
John Yudkin FRSC, 1910 – 1995, British physiologist and nutritionist, and the founding professor of the Department of Nutrition at Queen Elizabeth College, London, UK

Forty years of propaganda have given fat a bad name. There is not one jot of evidence for the risible theory that states high-fat diets cause high cholesterol and arterial disease. No! No! No!

In short, let fat be thy medicine and medicine be thy fat!
Dr Gabriela Segura, consultant cardiologist and cardiothoracic surgeon

All fats which occur *naturally* are good fats.

Saturated fats

In Nature there is no such thing as a bad fat. All are good. 'Bad' fats are man-made. We cannot easily destroy saturated fats. These medium-chain (8-18 carbon atoms) are tough, straight, stiff molecules in which every carbon atom is 'saturated', either with another carbon or with a hydrogen atom, and are solid at room temperature. Use lard (beef, pork or lamb), dripping, goose fat, butter, coconut oil or palm oil for cooking; when heated (which shakes things up) these retain their normal shape. Cocoa fat is also saturated. Fat is stored in our body as saturated fat and makes for a perfect pantry – essential fuel for lean times.

Lauric acid is just one such saturated fat and looks as shown in Figure 3.1 – straight, tough and stable.

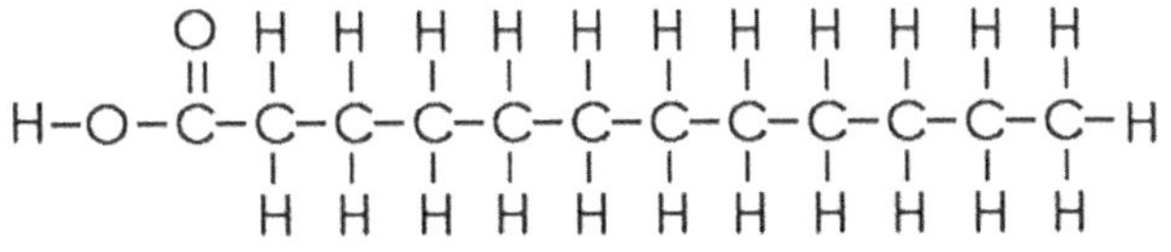

Figure 3.1: The structure of a saturated fat (lauric acid)

Unsaturated fats

Unsaturated fats are long-chain (20-26 carbon atoms) unsaturated, unstable, kinked molecules. The occasional hydrogen atom is 'missing' and so we get a double carbon bond instead which introduces a kink. If we have one double carbon bond, then we call this fat 'mono-unsaturated' (such as olive oil) and if we have more than one double carbon bond, we call these fats 'poly-unsaturated' (this includes most nut, seed, vegetable and fish oils). These double carbon bonds 'kink' the molecule and the molecule is named according to where it is kinked on the carbon chain – so for example we have omega-3, omega-6 and omega-9 (see Figure 3.2 for an example of how this 'kinking' may look).

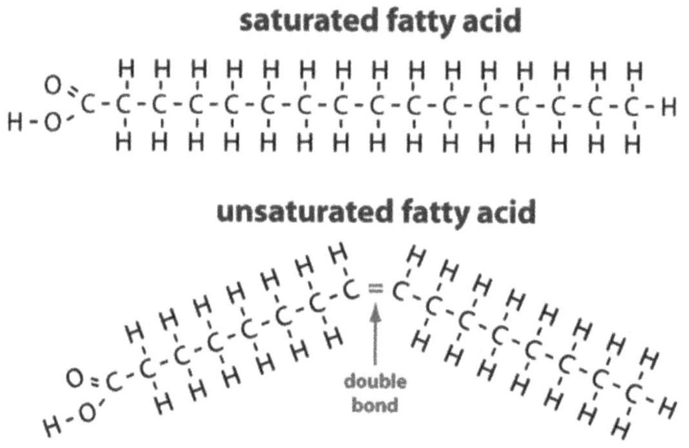

saturated fatty acid

unsaturated fatty acid

double
bond

Figure 3.2: The structure of a saturated fatty acid (palmitic acid) and an unsaturated fatty acid (palmitoleic acid), both with 16 carbon atoms

These fats we use as building materials, largely for membranes. Indeed, many biological actions take place on membranes, actions such as energy generation and nerve conduction. These fats are also called essential fatty acids because the body can't synthesise these oils for itself - they have to be eaten.

Trans-fats

In Nature, these kinks are all 'left-handed' and are called cis-fats. They fit our biochemistry perfectly. Problems arise when we heat (cook with) or hydrogenate (to make margarine and 'spreads') these fats. They flip into a right-handed version; these are what are called trans-fats. Just as a right hand will not fit into a left-handed glove, so trans-fats do not fit our biochemistry, and consequently they clog up our systems and are highly damaging. Figure 3.3 shows the problem: the trans-fat is not the same shape as the cis-fat.

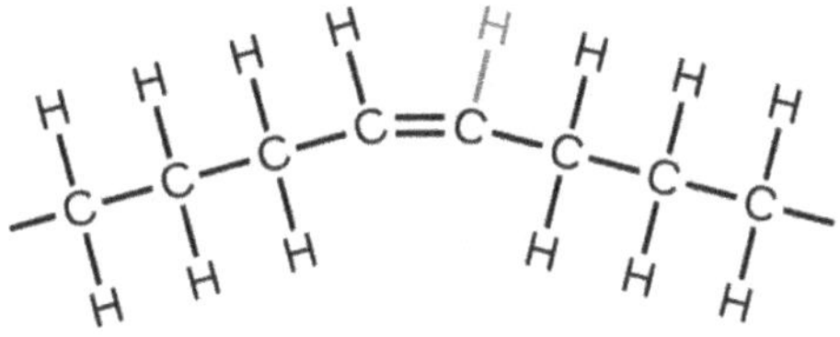

cis-fat molecule

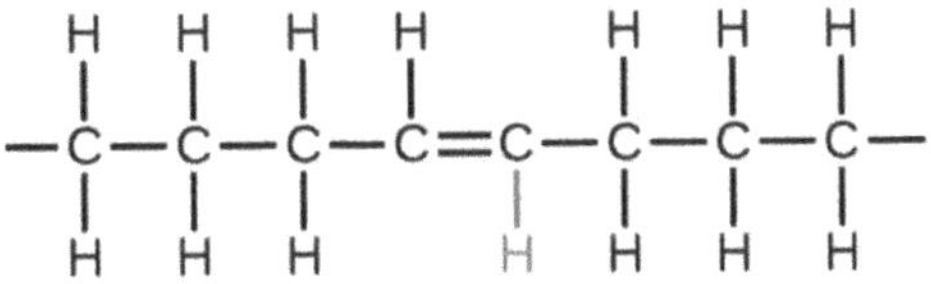

trans-fat molecule

Figure 3.3: Comparison of the structure of a natural unsaturated cis-fat with a man-made trans-fat

Which fats to eat

Knowing what we do, the rules of the game are:
- cook *only* with saturated fats such as lard (any animal fat), butter or coconut oil as these fats retain their shape after cooking.
- use oils, cold-pressed, *only* at room temperature – do not cook with them.
- do *not* eat hydrogenated fats (as in margarine) – if the fat has been hydrogenated, then the resulting trans-fat will not fit with your biochemistry.
- do *not* cook with unsaturated fats – No, it is not safe to cook with olive oil!

We are cautioned about the need for fat by the following English nursery rhyme, 'Jack Sprat' being an expression for people of small stature in 17th Century England. Mr Sprat was a weakling because:

> *Jack Sprat could eat no fat,*
> *His wife could eat no lean;*
> *And so between the two of them*
> *They licked the platter clean.* *

Carbohydrates

You may think I am maligning all carbohydrates. Not so; they are essential. Five-carbon sugars, such as D ribose, are the raw material to make ATP, DNA and RNA, the fundamental molecules of Life. Sugar is used to detoxify nasties in the liver via the process of glucuronidation. (NB: 10% of the population have lost this pathway and have a tendency to jaundice because they cannot detoxify bilirubin efficiently. This is called Gilbert's syndrome and sufferers are at greater risk of chronic fatigue syndrome because they are at risk of poisoning.) We have even evolved the ability to create sugar in the liver from protein via the process of gluconeogenesis. This reflects not only how essential sugar is, but also its rarity in primitive diets.

On the sporadic primitive occasion when there was an abundance of sugar, our wonderful metabolism allowed this to be shunted into use as a fuel or a fat – no waste there. Now all those eating a Western diet are awash with the stuff and it is poisoning us. As the classic toxicology maxim tells us, *Dosis sola facit venenum*, 'the dose makes the poison'.

> *All things are poison, and nothing is without poison; the dosage alone makes it so; a thing is not a poison.*
>
> Paracelsus[†], 1493 – 1541

---

* An early version of this rhyme appeared in John Clarke's collection of sayings in 1639.

[†] Ironically, Paracelsus died from chronic mercury intoxication as a late effect of his alchemical experiments.

40

We need to eat the right amount of carbohydrate – not so much that we overwhelm our gut's ability to digest it or our liver and muscle glycogen sponge to mop it up. Measuring ketones allows us to get the balance right (see Chapter 4).

Eat seasonally for variety

We know remarkably little about the gut microbiome, but we do know that the greater the variety of microbes within, the healthier we are. My guess is that within the gut, just as in Nature, there is an ecosystem with specific predator-prey interactions.[‡]

My guess is microbes too have favourite foods. Numbers increase exponentially when that food is present, when absent that microbe goes into hibernation. The greater the variety of foods eaten, the greater the diversity of microbes. One day we will know which food you need for each microbe. For example, we do know that friendly *E coli* thrive on the fibre in chickpeas, hazel nuts and figs. Products of such friendly fermentation include folic acid, vitamin K2, co-enzyme Q10 and the amino acids tyrosine and phenylalanine (these are precursors to dopamine, lack of which results in low mood) and tryptophan (a precursor to serotonin, the 'happy' neurotransmitter). This is just one example of over a thousand species of bacteria, up to a hundred species of fungi and about 140,000 different viruses known to populate the bowel. Like the universe, it's complicated.

> All you really need to know for the moment is that the universe is a lot more complicated than you might think, even if you start from a position of thinking it's pretty damn complicated in the first place.
>
> Douglas Adams, 11 March 1952 – 11 May 2001,
> *The Ultimate Hitchhiker's Guide to the Galaxy*

Eat vegetables, fruit, nuts and seeds that are in season. I am very fortunate to have a garden where seasonal food is the norm. As I write now in March, I am cooking red

---

[‡] **Mathematical aside:** predator-prey interactions are a topic in Mathematical Biology. It is all about relative rates of predation and reproduction; in a beautiful piece of mathematics, one can show what naturalists have known for centuries – that there is an equilibrium point between predator and prey where numbers of each remain stable. Of course, add in multiple prey and multiple predators and unexpected events (e.g. prey or predator-specific pathogens) and things become much more complicated and even more exciting! For the seriously interested, see Dr Ruth Baker's lecture notes.[2]

cabbage, Russian kale, cavolo nero, leeks, parsnip, Jerusalem artichokes and squash (stored) and eating raw cut-leaf parsley, coriander, land cress, winter lettuce, sage, marjoram, rosemary, rocket and onions, together with grated beetroot, carrot, kohl rabi, sauerkraut and hard pears from the outside store.

Bone broth: providing the raw materials for connective tissue

Friction between biological surfaces is damaging. It results in wear and tear which is painful and energy sapping. All moving machines use tricks to minimise friction, such as finely engineered weight-bearing surfaces, ball-bearings and lubricating oils. The body is no different and employs similar techniques to minimise friction. These include the ultra-smooth surfaces of joints, synovial lubricating fluid between joints, special pockets of such fluid to minimise friction of moving tendons (bursae), together with a softer matrix of fibrous/elastic material we call collagen. This is further steeped in a semi-solid colloidal, mucous matrix. Collectively we call this connective tissue. This is a terribly boring name for a divine conglomeration that allows our soft tissues to look gorgeous and function beautifully despite being suspended from an unforgiving, bone-hard skeleton.

Connective tissues are separated by a colloid gel which has just the right consistency to hold them together whilst at the same time allowing them to slide without friction. These colloid gels include joint fluid (synovial fluid), cerebrospinal fluid (in the brain), pleural fluid (in the lungs), peritoneal fluid (in the gut), tears, saliva and mucus. They include substances like hyaluronan and lubricin which have an amazing property described by one of my favourite words – they are thixotropic.[§] The fluids become more viscous under pressure. This further protects any weight-bearing surface. Additionally, these colloid gels become less viscous with movement, which explains why muscle

---

[§]**Linguistic and historical note:** The word 'thixotropy' derives from Ancient Greek -θίξις *thixis* 'touch' and τρόπος *tropos* 'of turning'. It was invented by Herbert Freundlich, originally for a sol-gel transformation. If the behaviour of fluids interests you, I am reliably informed by Craig that you should research Newtonian and non-Newtonian fluids.

[¶] **Linguistic and historical note:** The word 'brothel' derives from the Middle English 'broth', a worthless person, and is a stem of the word 'brethen' or *brēothan*, meaning to decay or degenerate. Rudyard Kipling is thought to have been the originator of the phrase 'the world's oldest profession'. His 1888 story, *On the City Wall*, about a prostitute, begins with the sentence, 'Lalun is a member of the most ancient profession in the world.'

stiffness can be helped by movement such as stretching or massage – this business of movement reduces the friction.

All the raw materials for reducing such frictions are freely available in bone broth (see the recipe on page 177) and this is an essential part of the PK kitchen. Weston Price, author of *Nutrition and Physical Degeneration* recommended brothels[¶] in every home!

> *What... we need... is healthy fast food and the only way to provide this is to put brothals in every town, independently owned brothals that provide the basic ingredient for soups and sauces and stews. And brothals will come when ... we... recognise that the food industry has prostituted itself to short cuts and huge profits, shortcuts that cheat consumers of the nutrients they should get in their food and profits that skew the economy towards industrialisation in farming and food processing.[3]*

Bone broth is the perfect food for:

- reducing connective tissue friction. Any friction from physical damage or inflammation (infection, allergy, autoimmunity) results in pain and disability. Examples include peritonitis, meningitis, pericarditis, pleurisy, periostitis, costochondritis, bursitis, neuritis, arteritis and tendonitis. Sufferers of these conditions will tell you that any movement results in severe pain because these movements are no longer without friction. Furthermore, the body's reaction to this friction is to prevent movement. This gives us the symptom of muscle stiffness. The starting point for treatment is bone broth.
- healing and repair of skin, blood vessels, tendons, muscles and nerve sheaths and the coverings of internal organs, including those of the gut (peritoneum), brain (meninges), heart (pericardium), lungs (pleural membranes) and bones (periosteum).
- supporting brains and immunity. Bone marrow and brains are especially rich in micronutrients. Large mammals invested huge amounts of energy and resources to develop powerful jaws to crack open bones to access this valuable resource. We can achieve the same by boiling bones. If you wish to have good quality bone marrow (to make blood and for the immune system), together with healthy nerves, you need the raw materials. All can be acquired from bone broth.
- repairing leaky gut. The gut wall is held together by connective tissue. Poor quality connective tissue may result in a leaky gut and all the associated problems. We seem to be seeing epidemics of hypermobility syndrome (EDS or Ehlers-Danlos

syndrome), often associated with chronic fatigue syndrome and, almost certainly, leaky gut.

- treating arthritis and osteoporosis. Bone broth contains all the raw materials for healthy bone – a host of essential minerals, such as calcium, magnesium, phosphorus, potassium, silicon, sulphur, selenium, zinc, boron, copper and manganese as well as essential building materials such as glycine, proline, arginine, various chondroitins, glucosamine, gelatine, hyaluronic acid and other such. Gelatine is abundant in bone broth and has a long history of excellence in the treatment of arthritis and osteoporosis. Twice-boiled chicken bones are an effective Chinese remedy for arthritis.
- building healthy skin, hair and nails. Bone broth contains the raw materials to make keratin. This is one of the toughest proteins in Nature. So many of my patients comment that the quality of their skin, hair and nails has been greatly improved by bone broth. Indeed, nail health reflects bone health and a good DIY test for osteo-porosis is to look at your nails. Hard, strong, tough-to-cut nails reflect hard, strong, hard-to-break bones. Improved skin quality is another bonus.

Timing

Primitive man did not eat three regular meals a day, neither did he snack. Consultant neurologist Dale Bredesen reverses dementia with a PK diet but insists all daily food is consumed within a 10-hour window of time.[4]

> *The best sauce is hunger.*
> This quotation is derived from *De finibus bonorum et malorum* ('On the ends of good and evil'), a philosophical work by Marcus Tullius Cicero, 106 BC – 43 BC, in which he also says *cibi condimentum esse famem* (hunger is the spice of food)

Once keto-adapted you may feel a bit peckish and deserving of a snack, but the good news is that you will not get the associated 'energy dive' experienced by the carb addict who must eat according to the clock. Carb addicts feel a sudden loss of energy and *have* to feed their addiction to get rid of this awful feeling. The keto-adapted do not experience this. A weekly 24-hour fast is also good for the metabolism. It may be counterintuitive, but the fact is that this enhances mental and physical performance (see Chapter 23).

Conclusion

Remember, none of the above are hard-and-fast rules. Listen to your body and follow your appetite. Once you are no longer addicted to foods, appetite is a remarkably good guide.

> *Variety is the very spice of life, that gives it all its flavour.*[#]
>
> William Cowper's poem *The Task*, 1785

Everyone is different; you are not a percentage.

> *Say you were standing with one foot in the oven and one foot in an ice bucket. According to the percentage people, you should be perfectly comfortable.*
>
> Bobby Bragan, 1963

Now you have the rules of the game and the tools of the trade but, like cricket, you must develop your own style. Geoffrey Boycott and Ian Botham both followed the rules of the game (mostly!) and both played very well (mostly) and yet they were very different players with idiosyncratic styles of play. So for how to get started… read on.

> *In politics, if you want anything said, ask a man; if you want anything done, ask a woman.*
>
> Margaret Thatcher as MP for Finchley in 1965

[#] When Craig was a young boy, he would often act as waiter at the parties his mum and dad would throw. Craig was effectively an only child from the age of 7 because his brother went to boarding school. The same boarding place was offered to Craig but, because he had witnessed his mother cry the whole journey home after dropping his brother off at school for the first term away, he simply refused to leave home, preferring instead the local state grammar school. Anyway, Craig would earwig at these parties and learnt much. In response to someone quoting 'Variety is the spice of life', a partygoer, who had been married three times and whose grammar was somewhat amiss, mistaking spice for the plural of spouse, retorted: 'No, no! Spice is the variety of life!'

Chapter 4

Getting started

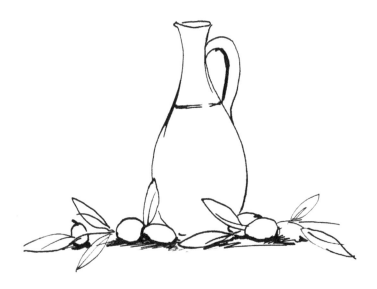

In order to get from A to B, you first have to leave A.
$\qquad$ Craig's father on numerous occasions

So, you have to commit, and then you have to start:
- First sort out your pantry (chuck out the temptations) and stock your fridge and freezer (see Chapter 6: The PK pantry).
- Learn to make PK bread (see Chapter 8, page 82).
- Purchase a ketone breath meter.

- Allocate a window of time when you are not socialising (if possible, buddy up with another who is going PK)
- Then just do it

Knowing you are in ketosis

You can determine that you are in ketosis by using a ketone breath meter, plus being aware of the symptoms and signs. Ketones arise through burning fat, which generates three types of ketone which can be monitored in different ways:

- Beta hydroxybutyric acid, present in, and which can be measured in, the blood – this is the most accurate measure, but testing strips are expensive. I am mean and a wimp, so I do not use this method.
- Acetoacetate is excreted in the urine. Testing is cheap and easy with urine keto-stix but as the body becomes more efficient at matching ketone production to demand, urine tests may show false negatives.
- Acetone is exhaled and can be measured with breath testing. This is my preferred method and the one I recommend here as you can easily test after every meal to ensure you have not overdone the carbs.

You must test because everyone is different; there is no 'one size fits all' guidance here. Craig can eat 90 grams of carbs a day and happily stay in ketosis whereas I have to stick to 30 grams or less a day. Dammit! Men normally move into ketosis more easily than women because they have a higher metabolic rate, furthermore women have female sex hormones which are conducive to metabolic syndrome.

- No ketones on breath testing means we are running purely on sugars. This is not desirable in the long term.
- Low ketones on breath testing means we are burning some fats. This tells us our glycogen stores are not saturated and blood sugar levels will be completely stable. This is a very desirable state of affairs.

What this means in practice is that the occasional seasonal excursion into autumn delights, when we slip out of ketosis, will do little harm to our health. 'Autumn mode' is fine in the short term but damaging to health in the long term. Long-term 'autumn mode' results in metabolic syndrome. I like to see my patients blowing ketones at least once a day, which tells me their glycogen stores are not saturated. A common pattern is no ketones in the morning (when blood sugar levels are naturally higher) but by late afternoon or evening, ketones are present. Being in constant ketosis is absolutely fine but some people feel better with a little more carb in their diet.

Once you have established a state of ketosis, checked by testing, you will learn to 'recognise' when you are in ketosis and will 'know' when you have kicked yourself out of it too. I know if I slip out of ketosis because I start thinking about my next meal. In ketosis I often forget lunch. Craig, for example, knows when he is out of ketosis because mental sharpness declines dramatically and then, once back into ketosis, he can think with clarity again – it is almost like an electric buzz in his brain. We all have our own individual signs of being in ketosis and you will come to recognise yours.

Trouble-shooting the ketone breath test

What to expect normally
If your diet is sufficiently low-carb, expect to blow 2-6 parts per million (ppm) of ketones. However, the body will always use sugar in preference to ketones. This means that *any* amount of ketones in the breath signifies that you are in ketosis.

If you blow very high levels of ketones (e.g. up to 10 ppm), this may be because:
*   when stressed, there is an outpouring of adrenalin and this stimulates fat burning.
*   you are fasting. Even on a PK diet you consume some carbohydrates. With fasting you get *all* your calories from fat, so ketones are higher. This illustrates the point that even in mild ketosis you will be using some sugars as a fuel – that is fine.
*   over-dosing with thyroid hormones may cause high levels of ketones.
*   contamination as below.

Possible problem results
False positives: You can get false positive results for a number of reasons. The mechanism used to measure ketones is the same as that for measuring alcohol. You may therefore see a positive:
*   if you have consumed any alcohol in the past 24 hours (depending on how much).
*   if you have a fermenting upper gut, then this too produces alcohol.

Any products containing alcohol may give a positive result; I checked this myself with an alcohol wipe (often used for hand sanitising) to clean the mouthpiece and this gave a high reading, so watch out!

In addition, the meter measures parts per million; it is very sensitive. You need only a tiny amount of contaminant to upset the result. Many household cleaners contain volatile organic compounds which may register on the meter.

False negatives: You can also get false negative results. If you have anything to eat or drink, other than water, in the preceding 20 minutes then that may affect the test. For example, I know if I have a sip of coffee then that may be followed by a negative reading.

Breath ketone levels may not square with blood levels. This does not matter. They may also not square with urine ketones. It is not unusual to see ketones present on a breath test, but the urine test be negative. With time, the body gets better at matching energy demands to delivery, so fewer ketones are 'wasted' through urinary losses.

When ketosis is a problem

Being in ketosis is *not* dangerous. Most doctors do not know or understand physiological ketosis. They only know about diabetic ketoacidosis and may panic if you tell them you are in ketosis.

Ketosis is a medical problem *only* if you are diabetic and your blood sugars are running high (either because your medication is insufficient OR because you are consuming too many carbs). For example, a blood sugar reading above 10 mmol/l and/or the presence of sugar in your urine are signs that, yes, this is a *medical emergency*.

At the same time, bear in mind that the DIY home tests for blood sugar rely on a process that employs glucose oxidase. Vitamin C cross-reacts, so if you are taking vitamin C to bowel tolerance your blood will be saturated with vitamin C and this may give false highs. You can test for this with urine dip-sticks that measure vitamin C. My experience is that the DIY blood sugar measurements may be 2-3 mmol/l higher than the actual blood glucose level. That is to say, an apparent reading of 7-8 mmol/l equates to a real reading of 4-5 mmol of glucose. If there is any doubt, then trot down to your GP for a laboratory test.

The benefits of being in ketosis

As you get into ketosis you will benefit from some or all of the changes listed in Table 4.1.

Table 4.1: What to expect when getting into ketosis

What	Why
In the short term after 1-2 weeks	It takes some days to burn up your saturated glycogen stores and switch into ketosis
Energy levels improve	Mitochondria run more efficiently on ketones. The heart and brain run up to 25% more efficiently burning ketones compared with sugar (see our book *Diagnosis and Treatment of Chronic Fatigue Syndrome and Myalgic Encephalitis – it's mitochondria not hypochondria*). Once keto-adapted the blood sugar level can run as low as 1 pmol/l without symptoms of hypoglycaemia arising
Mental performance is improved	The preferred fuel for the brain is ketones. The newborn baby runs entirely on ketones with the brain using 60% of all energy production. The ketogenic diet is the starting point to treat all brain pathologies from mental disease and dementia to epilepsy and malignant tumours
Physical and mental endurance ability is better	The glycogen pantry lasts for only 1700 Kcal (about 16 miles for marathon runners at which point they 'hit a wall'; US athletes call this 'bonking'). The fat pantry, even in a lean athlete, can last 140,000 Kcal. The world record for the furthest distance run in 24 hours is held by keto-adapted athlete Mike Morton. He ran 172 miles
	Dr Ian Lake, GP and type 1 diabetic, with seven friends ran 100 miles in five days from Henley to Bristol between 19 and 23 September 2020 whilst fasting
You stop constantly thinking and obsessing about food	There is a constant and reliable fuel available to the body. The brain is not consumed by that next carb fix
Blood sugar levels stabilise because the body is burning fat	Levels of insulin and adrenalin remain constant. (Adrenalin spikes as blood sugars fall in someone not keto-adapted – low blood sugar 'hypoglycaemia' symptoms are largely adrenalin symptoms (see Chapter 5: The metabolic hinterland)

What	Why
You feel calmer once in established ketosis – mood swings greatly reduce	I suspect the symptom of stress arises when the brain knows it does not have the physical, mental or emotional energy to deal with Life's challenges. Being in ketosis increases the energy available in all departments. A ketogenic diet also increases levels of the calming neurotransmitter, GABA
You can miss a meal without getting an energy dive	One can survive on fat burning for weeks (depending on the size of your fat store). Indeed, periods of fasting stimulate new brain neurones to grow and this makes us cleverer (see Chapter 23)
Sleep quality is better – you may need fewer hours of sleep	The commonest cause of disturbed and poor-quality sleep is nocturnal hypoglycaemia because of the adrenalin spike associated with such. Perhaps the next commonest cause is snoring due to obesity, then allergy, typically to dairy products
You may lose 1-2 kilos of weight very quickly	Carbohydrates are stored in the liver and muscle as glycogen. This has an osmotic pressure – i.e. it holds water. Once glycogen is used up prior to fat burning this water is peed out. This is one reason why endurance athletes see a rapid improvement in performance—the power-weight ratio is instantly improved
You cure your fermenting mouth and stop dental decay. Teeth become glassy smooth	Dental plaque gives teeth a rough surface. Dental plaque is the biofilm behind which teeth-rotting bacteria (*Streptococcus mutans*) hide. These microbes can ferment sugar and starches only. The ketogenic diet starves them out. Dental decay ceases. Halitosis is often cured (it may also derive from the fermenting gut and/or airway infections (chest, throat and sinuses))
Clean tongue	Tongues become dirty and discoloured because of bacterial colonies sticking to and fermenting on them; they should be pink and free from surface crud. Gum disease (gingivitis) is driven by sugar and starches. You can speed this process up by gargling with hydrogen peroxide 3% mouthwash
You cure your fermenting upper gut	This is because you deprive those fermenters of substrate. Symptoms of burping, reflux, acidity, indigestion, bloating, pain and irritable bowel disappear. You greatly reduce your risk of bowel disease, from inflammatory bowel and gallbladder disease to diverticulitis and cancer

In the longer term – months to years	
You cure metabolic syndrome and reverse diabetes	This is because you stabilise blood sugar levels and reverse insulin resistance. Blood pressure comes down. You correct your cholesterol. (For much more detail see out books *Prevent and Cure Diabetes* and *Ecological Medicine*)
You improve immune function	All microbes love sugar. Metabolic syndrome is a major risk factor for infection including covid-19. (For much more detail see our book *The Infection Game: life is an arms race*)
You alleviate any problem associated with inflammation	The ketogenic diet is anti-inflammatory. Furthermore, many conditions I suspect are driven by allergy to gut microbes. These include polymyalgia rheumatica, many arthritides (e.g. rheumatoid arthritis, ankylosing spondylitis), venous ulcers, autoimmune conditions, intrinsic asthma, psoriasis, chronic urticaria, interstitial cystitis, many psychiatric conditions, inflammatory bowel disease and nephritis as well as many other possibilities. (See our book *Ecological Medicine*)
The quality of your skin and mucous membranes improves	High-fat diets improve the quality of skin and mucous membranes. Dry skin, dry eyes, dry mouth and dry perineums (vulva and vagina) may result from low fat diets

The unexpectedly complicated journey

And we leave you with a mathematical aside, known as the Speed Paradox, about getting from A to B (and back again). You can watch Dr Robin Wilson (former tutor of Craig, and son of the Prime Minister, Harold Wilson) describe it here: www.youtube.com/watch?v=ZIO-ExZVkdw or you can see it laid out as follows:

You drive from Oxford to Cambridge at 40 mph.
You then drive from Cambridge to Oxford at 60 mph.
What is your average speed for the entire journey?
Many people say 50 mph, but they are wrong!
The actual answer is 48 mph.

And this works for any journey between any two places where one travels one way at 40 mph and the other at 60 mph.

The maths

Here are the calculations, with the distance from Oxford to Cambridge being d miles, though it is actually irrelevant what the distance is. Then we use these equations:

Speed = Distance DIVIDED by Time

and

Time = Distance DIVIDED by Speed

So, the time taken to drive from Oxford to Cambridge is

Distance (d) DIVIDED by Speed (40) = d/40

and the time taken to drive from Cambridge to Oxford is

Distance (d) DIVIDED by Speed (60) = d/60

So, the total time taken is

d/40 PLUS d/60 = 6d/240 PLUS 4d/240 = 10d/240 = d/24

And you have driven a distance of 2d – that is, from Oxford to Cambridge and back again – so, your average speed is

Distance (2d) DIVIDED by Time (d/24) or 48 mph.

The lesson

This just goes to show that journeys can be more complex than you first thought, so be prepared but do stick with it. It is worth it, as Craig and I can attest. *Just do it!*

Chapter 5

Troubleshooting: Diet, detox and die-off (DDD) reactions

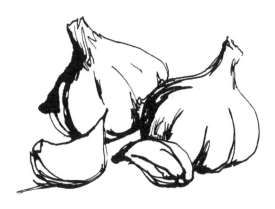

If I do not actively warn my patients of the likelihood of diet, detox and die-off reactions then I can expect an anxious email or telephone call. The sicker you are, the worse you can expect these reactions to be. You may have to go into the regimes gently and slowly, but go you must. Again, you have first to leave A in order to get to B. Either way, it is not fun. Try to see these reactions as a good sign that you are on the right path. You will need a good sense of humour.

Diet reactions

There are three common players: the metabolic hinterland, addiction reactions and allergy.

1. The metabolic hinterland

The transition from burning carbs to burning fat is difficult and takes time – usually 1-2 weeks. The body has been used to running on carbs and there is an inertia in the system; it is as if it takes time to 'learn' fat burning. During this window of time the body cannot get fuel from carbs (because they have been cut out of the diet) so it uses adrenalin to burn fat. To the patient this gives some of the symptoms of low blood sugar because adrenalin is partly responsible for such. We call this 'keto flu' but it has also been given the dreadful and confusing name 'ketogenic hypoglycaemia'. It was first described in the 1960s in children treated for epilepsy with a ketogenic diet. Let me explain further.

We have the collective symptoms of low blood sugar for reasons of low blood sugar *and* the hormonal responses to this situation:

- Poor energy delivery due to low blood sugar: fatigue, foggy brain and, potentially, loss of consciousness (which is why diabetics on medication *must* closely monitor their blood sugar).
- Adrenalin release: feeling 'hyper', shaky, anxious, possibly with palpitations and fast heart rate.
- Gut hormone responses: feelings of hunger and the need to eat.

If all is well with your metabolism, your body switches into fat burning (and it takes 1-2 weeks for this to happen, as I have said) and all the above symptoms, which we associate with low blood sugar, disappear.

If all is not well with your metabolism, then these symptoms do not disappear and the clinical picture which results is so-called 'keto-flu' or 'ketogenic hypoglycaemia'. It is characterised by:

- Blood sugar levels are normal or (even better) low and stable.
- You are in ketosis (confirmed by blood, urine or breath tests).
- BUT you continue to have those nasty adrenalin symptoms of being 'hyper', shaky, anxious, possibly with palpitations and fast heart rate.
- You continue to suffer the gut hormone symptoms of intense hunger and the need to eat.
- So clinically this feels exactly like hypoglycaemia.

There are three common causes:

1. Time: Some people just take time to keto-adapt – the body has to 'learn' fat

burning, but there are also emotional and psychological reasons why it is hard to change the habits of a lifetime.

2. Lack of carnitine: This is the short-chain polypeptide which is essential for transporting ketones into mitochondria. Carnitine works like the fuel injectors of engines. As its name implies, it is derived from meat. Vegetarians and vegans may wallow in the metabolic hinterland because of lack of carnitine. It can be corrected reliably well with acetyl L carnitine 0.5-2 grams daily.

3. Hypothyroidism: The body normally switches into fat burning by using thyroid hormones. If these are insufficient then it will use adrenalin instead and this gives us the symptoms of hypoglycaemia. To sort this, see our book *Ecological Medicine*. This problem is very common and often is unmasked in women at the menopause.

The journey through this 'metabolic hinterland' must become your personal crusade, indeed your Pilgrim's Progress. Craig and I have done it and can now smile smugly from a ketogenic heaven. But at least Craig and I are cheering you on from the other side… so read on and be encouraged.

In summary, the metabolic hinterland is characterised by:

*   Lack of fuel (either carbohydrates or fats) for the body to burn. This results in horrible symptoms of fatigue, feeling cold, foggy brain and depression.
*   The temptation to go for instant relief of these ghastly symptoms by eating carbohydrates, such as a banana.
*   But this spikes insulin.
*   An hour later on we again find ourselves in the metabolic hinterland with the worst of both worlds – the banana fuel has run out and the insulin spike means one cannot burn fat for some hours. Back to the fatigue, the freezer, the fog and the funk hole.
*   The overwhelming temptation, which subverts all else, is to eat another banana … and so it goes on, just like the drug addict!

This explains why so many struggle initially with the PK diet. They start off by cutting down on carbohydrates instead of drastically reducing them. They drop into the metabolic hinterland and get stuck there, lethargic, foggy, cold and depressed. Instant relief is a banana away, short-term temptation prevails, and they slip back into metabolic syndrome. We must be better than Oscar Wilde when he said: 'I can resist anything except temptation'

2. Addiction reactions

We use addiction to mask unpleasant symptoms such as fatigue, foggy brain or pain. Stop the addiction and those symptoms return. Ghastly in the short term, great in the long. Obviously addiction to sugar and starch is illustrated by the metabolic hinterland, but chocolate, caffeine, alcohol, nicotine, cola and other such all have the potential to cause withdrawal or 'train spotting' pains, inflammations and fatigue. And yes, I love caffeine but have it in small doses.* It is best to use this mid-morning – you should be at you best early morning (so not need it) and as caffeine has a long half-life with the potential to disrupt sleep, have none after midday.

3. Allergy reactions

Allergy and addiction are two sides of the same coin. I once had a patient who, before I was allowed to speak, declared that when he died, he would like to take a cow to heaven with him to ensure a supply of his favourite food. The diagnosis was not difficult. He was cured by cutting out dairy products. The point here is that if you love and are drawn to a particular food, think allergy. Stopping allergy foods in the short term may cause similar withdrawal symptoms as above.

Detoxification reactions

In the short term the body can deal with a spike of some toxic load by stuffing these toxins into fat. When I do fat biopsies (and I have yet to see a normal result of zero) results come back in milligrams per kilogram. By contrast, blood results come back in micrograms per kilogram. This alone tells us toxic levels in fat are a thousand-fold higher than in blood.

Losing weight and/or mobilising fat is/are intrinsic to a ketogenic diet. This may mobilise toxins from fat into the bloodstream and cause an acute poisoning. The improved nutrition of multivitamins, minerals, essential fatty acids and vitamin C has

---

* **Footnote re caffeine from Craig:** Sarah is not alone in her love of caffeine. I drink green tea every day and I make a cup of coffee for my wife, Penny, first thing in the morning every day too. According to Fulgoni et al (2015) 89% of Americans consume some caffeine every day of their lives.

a similar effect. Mobilising such chemicals is akin to throwing a handful of sand into a finely tuned engine and may produce almost any symptom (see below). In the very short term, energy delivery mechanism will be impaired. Many toxic metals and chemicals are immunotoxic – that is, they switch on inflammation. In short, there may be a temporary poisoning. Again, this is bad in the short term but good in the long. (There is much more detail in our comprehensive book *Ecological Medicine*.)

Die-off (Herx) reactions

Die-off reactions were first described by two immunologists, Drs Jarisch and Herxheimer, in patients with syphilis treated with antimicrobials and are consequently known as a 'Herxheimer response' or 'Herx'. It is partly due to endotoxin-like products released by the death of micro-organisms within the body and partly to immune activation. (I think of this as 'allergy to dead microbes').

Greatly reducing carbohydrates in the diet and using vitamin C to bowel tolerance will kill off many unfriendly microbes fermenting in the upper gut, and perhaps elsewhere, with the potential to trigger a Herx. Again, this is short-term pain but long-term gain.

DDD symptoms

DDD reactions may cause any symptom. The sicker you are when starting the regimes, the more likely you are to suffer DDD reactions. This presents a great problem to the clinician and patient alike because some are so sick they cannot afford to get much worse. It is always a precarious balancing act.

Those symptoms may be:
- Worsening of current symptoms.
- Inflammation:
  - o systemic symptoms (fever, malaise, aches and pains, depression, flu-like symptoms and sickness behaviour) or
  - o local (acute cold, cough, catarrh, diarrhoea, cystitis etc) (see our book *Ecological Medicine*).
- Poor energy delivery mechanisms: fatigue, foggy brain, low mood and depression.

Principles of treatment of DDD reactions

There are various ways to manage DDD reactions:
- Try to work out the cause and address it specifically.
- Temporarily relax the regimes: wean yourself off your addictions over time and introduce the regimes more slowly. This goes against our Golden Rule of 'just one biscuit being the road to disaster' (Chapter 2) *but* in cases where DDD reactions are troublesome, one has to be pragmatic.
- Give it time: Time is a vital part of the diagnostic and therapeutic process. An initial consultation with me usually concludes: 'You may love me now but in a week's time you will hate me.' It is no consolation to tell them that I too have been on the same journey and been equally grumpy about the whole process… I am sure Craig has experienced the same.[†]

> *Don't be afraid to take a big step if one is indicated. You can't cross a chasm in two small jumps.*
> David Lloyd George, 17 January 1863 – 26 March 1945, British politician

- Expect a bumpy ride: These reactions do not follow a smooth course.

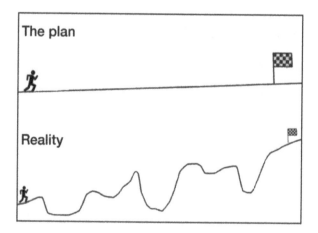

[†] Gentleman Craig replies: 'Indeed, I have but I have never "hated" Sarah! When going through these DDD reactions, I have always had Penny on hand to remind me, "This is just what Sarah said might happen!".'

The darkest hour is before dawn.

Old English Proverb now universally used

The longer term

Once established on the PK diet …however you are …stick with it for Life!

The word 'doctor' comes from the Latin to teach. I can show you the path, but you have to walk it. You have to become your own doctor. All diagnosis starts with hypothesis. We know the PK diet is the starting point to treat every disease and that this is non-negotiable. Stick with this diet for life and it may be that this is all you have to do. Once it is established you have to ask if you are functioning to your full physical and mental potential? Only you can know this.

If you reckon you are, then you can really enjoy the occasional feast (see Chapter 20).

Even if you are not yet, you must stick with the PK diet. This diet is the foundation stone on which your recovery is built. If you are stuck, then move on to other interventions which can be found in our book *Ecological Medicine*. Even if you do not experience immediate benefits you will greatly increase your chance of a long and healthy life. It is a great consolation for me to be able to tell my CFS and ME patients that their best years are ahead of them.

The Chinese do not draw any distinction between food and medicine.
Lin Yutang, 1895 – 1976, Chinese writer in *The importance of Living*
chapter 9, section 7

Part II

The How

Recipes – the delicious practical reality from everyday staples to the PK gourmet

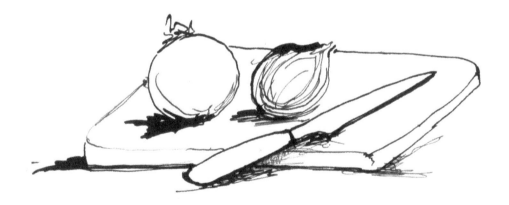

Chapter 6

The PK pantry

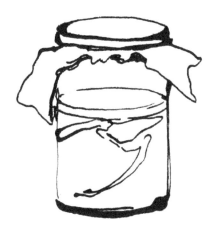

The word 'pantry' derives from the same source as the Old French term *paneterie* - that is, from *pain*, the French form of the Latin *panis*, 'bread', and a pantry was where bread was stored. In the late Middle Ages; the head of the pantry was called the *pantier*, and there were similar rooms for the storage of bacon and other meats (larder), and of alcoholic beverages (buttery – so called for the 'butts' of barrels stored there), and for cooking (kitchen). Some readers may have a pantry (now for the use of storing all food at a cool temperature) but for most of us here, the 'pantry' denotes where we store our food – cupboards, fridge, deep freeze, etc.

Use what follows as a shopping list. I have detailed foods in order of priority in my kitchen.

Cupboards

Grain substitutes: golden linseeds (whole), desiccated coconut, coconut flour

Seeds: sunflower, pumpkin, sesame, chia

Eggs

Nuts: Brazils, almonds, flaked coconut (I dare not store cashews because I get addicted to them)

Tinned fish: anchovies, sardines, mackerel, prawns, mussels, crab

Tinned meat: corned beef, paté, ham

Tinned tomatoes

Coconut cream (long-life e.g Grace)

Herbs: garlic, rosemary, thyme, coriander, basil

Pickles: gherkins, jalapeños

Spices: pepper, cumin, cardamon, cinnamon, ginger, nutmeg

Dried veg: tomatoes, peppers

Some dried fruit e.g. apple, apricot

Olives

Lemons

Avocados

Oils: cold-pressed hemp and olive oils; coconut oil

Mustard

Sunflower lecithin liquid

Balsamic vinegar

Coffee

Tea and herbal teas*

Dark chocolate 85% or more

Sunshine salt

Multivitamins

Vitamin C as ascorbic acid

Vitamin D 10,000 iu capsules

* **Note from Craig:** I can attest to the quality of the green tea.

Fridge

Vegan block butter (Naturali)
Butter or ghee (if you are sure you are not dairy-allergic)
Vegan cheeses
Coyo yoghurt
Lard, dripping, goose fat
Salami
Pate – liver, pork, brawn
Salad stuff (whatever is not in the garden)
Vegetables (whatever is in season or not in the garden; if you are not a gardener, then arrange for an organic-box vegetable delivery)
Mushrooms
Sauerkraut
Coleslaw
Ginger

Deep freeze

Joints of pork, chicken, lamb, beef, duck, fish
Sausage, beefburger, chops, mince, belly
Liver, hearts, kidneys
Leaf fat
Bones
Vegetables: garden gluts – broad beans, French beans
Berries: blackcurrants, gooseberries, raspberries, blueberries.

Garden

Whatever is in season – Cripes, I can feel a gardening book coming on!
Herbs: these are the first crops to plant; they are easy to grow, perennial (or
self-seed readily) and enhance any dish. My favourites are peppermint, sage,
rosemary,[†] land cress, parsley, coriander, rocket and horseradish.

Equipment

Over and above the usual:
Nutribullet grinder – essential for the fresh grinding of seeds
Slow cooker – for bone broth (page xx)
Spiraliser – for salads and coleslaws
Dehydrator – for garden gluts
A dog – for that canine pre-wash!
Two half-sized dishwashers – one for the dirty loading, one clean for current use.
That way you do not waste time or energy unloading and stashing kitchen imple-
ments. Crocks and cutlery can live permanently in the dishwasher.

Cooking equipment must be safe. We all remember the phase when we threw out our
aluminium cooking pans and replaced them with stainless steel. Miserably, stainless steel
is 14% nickel. Nickel is a major sensitising metal for switching on allergy and is a known
carcinogen.

I am in the throes of auditing all the toxicity tests which I do; these include DNA
adducts. This is a test for substances stuck on to DNA. Of course, there should be

---

[†] **Historical aside:** I am reminded of the lyrics of *Scarborough Fair*. Alternative refrains abound but I learnt the
'parsley, sage, rosemary and thyme' version. This ballad is a story of unrequited love and in its traditional form
has a man and woman singing alternate sections. A young man requests impossible tasks from his lover, saying
that if she can perform them, he will take her back. In return, she requests impossible things of him, saying she
will perform her tasks when he performs his. So, for example, he asks her to wash a shirt in a dry well that has
never sprung water and she replies with requiring him to find an acre of land between the salt water and the
sea sand. It regained prominence after the Simon and Garfunkel version, but my favourite version is sung by
Amy Nuttall (see YouTube), although in this version all the impossible tasks are set by the woman for the man.
(Quite right too! Craig.)

nothing. DNA should be pristine. Nickel is one of the commonest adducts so do not use stainless steel cookware. The next most frequent adducts are dyes (from food and hair colourants) and flame retardants from soft furnishings.

Non-stick is worse – it releases perfluoro-octanic acid with all the problems of fluoride. Copper cookware is not too bad, but acidic foods will leach copper out freely. Use pots and pans made from cast iron, pyrex, enamel, ceramic or stone.

For mixing I use pottery or hard ancient plastic (mine have had 60 years to outgas… yes, yes they are Mother's hand-me-downs).

The best fats you can buy

Lard and meat fat are inexpensive saturated fats, but they do vary greatly as regards quality. The quality of the lard is determined by the life of the animal. Lard from free-range, grass-fed, organic, mature animals will be far superior to that from intensively reared animals. It is worth putting much effort into establishing a great source of lard. I am so fortunate in having free-range pigs who can supply me.[‡]

It is always worth considering what was an animal was fed. 'You are what you eat' applies to animals as well as homo sapiens. On what was the animal fed? Pigs fed on fish meal taste of fish. These pigs have to be swapped to a grain-based diet for at least two weeks before slaughter. Where I live in Radnorshire all sheep and beef-cattle live free range on the hills. Their fat is always delicious.

> *Dis-moi ce que tu manges, je te dirai ce que tu es.*
> *[Tell me what you eat and I will tell you what you are.]*
> Anthelme Brillat-Savarin, 1 April 1755 – 2 February 1826, French lawyer and politician, and later an epicure and gastronome *Physiologie du Gout, ou Meditations de Gastronomie Transcendante*, 1826

[‡] **Note from Craig:** I have never seen (actually heard – see next sentence!) such happy pigs as those residing at Upper Weston. They are constantly oinking; scientists from the Universities of Lincoln and Belfast studied 72 male and female juvenile pigs and concluded that happier pigs and those with more curious temperaments grunt and squeal more than their less happy, less curious cousins.[3]

The best fat to buy is leaf (peritoneal, gut) or kidney fat. (The peritoneum is a layer of thin tissue that lines the abdomen and covers all of the organs within it, such as the bowel and the liver.) Professor Caroline Pond in her book *The Fats of Life* details how fat is laid down where the immune system is busy. This makes perfect evolutionary sense – the immune system is greatly demanding of energy and micronutrients; all these commodities need to be readily available for when the immune system is challenged. Furthermore, taste evolved for very good reasons – it allows us to select the most nutritious foods (see Chapter 16: Human pharmacognosy).

It is no co-incidence that 90% of the immune system is associated with the gut (the gut is heaving with microbes) and peritoneal, gut or leaf fat has the best flavour. Indeed, when I go to the butcher's,§ I ask for the lumpy leaf fat. Because it is not attractive, either physically or socially, I am often asked if I want it to feed the birds. 'Oh yes,' say I, thinking that the old buzzard standing in front of the gorgeous young butcher is to be the main recipient!

§ **Note from Craig:** Butchers are most often great sports and happy to educate townies like me. When Penny and I moved to our first house – a former miner's cottage in Pucklechurch (meaning 'Beautiful Church', from the Latin *'pulchra'* and where we were married) – we bought our meat from the local butcher. At the first visit introductions were made and the butcher said that he always gave a free chop to each new customer, and with that he spun round, took hold of a large cleaver, and there followed two large slamming noises and a scream. He turned round with blood eschewing and what seemed to be a thumb missing. Penny screamed, I turned this way and then that way, looking for I know not what. And then the butcher laughed: 'Got you there!' showing us the tomato ketchup and fake thumb. Apparently, he did this to all newcomers. However, we were happy – we had a new friend and two free chops. What more could we ask?

Chapter 7

Meals for those challenged
by energy, time and/or inclination

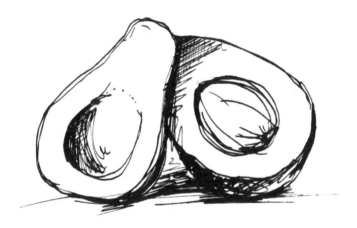

Some readers may be tempted to skip this chapter, which is primarily designed for the severely fatigued who are unable to cook meals for themselves and require carers to shop and cook for them. However, there will be occasions when you do not have the time or the inclination to prepare food and you need just to grab and eat. Start by stocking your pantry as described in the previous chapter. Then, follow the guidance and shopping lists below.

Meal suggestions

You may at first think this makes for a boring diet, but, as I say to my patients, 'My job is to get you well, not to entertain you'. As you recover you will then have the energy to move on to recipes, and the first recipe you must make is the PK bread (see page 82).

Table 7.1: Possible PK foods that require minimal preparation

Meal		Notes
Breakfast	Cocos yoghurt	Mix in ground linseed; adjust the amount to prevent constipation.
	Soya yoghurt, plain e.g. Alpro, Provamel	Mix in frozen berries from the deep freeze
	Cocos vanilla yoghurt 125 g	Ditto
Lunch and supper/ Starters	2 x avocado pears, mayonnaise, French dressing Slices salami, Parma ham, cold meat Tinned meat, fish, shellfish Celery stick with paté or vegan cheese Coleslaw Sauerkraut, pickled gherkins Tinned vegetable low-carb soup – stir in a dollop of coconut cream to give it substance	
	Coconut paleo wraps – expensive but delicious ... use sparingly	Care!... a single 14 g wrap contains 3 g of carbohydrate
Main course	Cold meat – ham, chicken etc Tinned fish or shellfish Tinned fish or shellfish Tinned meat Smoked mackerel fillets Tofu or quorn with pesto Washed salad – just open the package!	
Puddings	Cocos yoghurt, soya yoghurt Berries (fresh or frozen) with large dollop of Grace coconut milk	If still hungry drink the Grace coconut milk. This is my favourite coconut milk with just 2% carbs. Insist on the carton which for some odd reason is far superior to the tinned.

Snacks	Pork scratchings Olives 85% dark chocolate Brazil nuts, pecans, flaked coconut Spoonful of nut butter (eat off the spoon) Biltong	Always count the carbs of nuts and nut butters because it is easy to overdo them – see Appendix 1 for a guide. Check you are in ketosis with your ketone breath meter

The seven-day meal plan below ('Shopping list by meals for one week') is not intended to be prescriptive (everybody is different). As I have said, it is primarily for the severely disabled and/or for those people who are otherwise challenged by energy, time and/or inclination or those who need a 'quick-fix' PK meal-plan for a few days. For some people it may help to give them an idea of how they might initially approach a paleo-ketogenic way of eating so that they can easily get started. Don't stick to it in the long term or you will get bored and that is often a cause of failure.

This plan demonstrates that the paleo-ketogenic diet can be followed even if the individual is suffering severe disability. The idea is to provide a list of meal and food suggestions that require no preparation or cooking. In essence, this can be a temporary measure until you can cook more independently or until you have more time, and so don't think that this will have to be your diet forever. In fact, following this diet will give you more energy so that you become more able to cook independently and enjoy the other meals described later in this book.

Some people will need to go through this initial 'no cooking and no preparation' stage before they are able to move on to the delicious recipes found in the rest of the book, whereas some people will be able to 'skip' straight to those more appealing recipes without first going through this 'no cooking and no preparation' stage. However, the meal ideas here may be useful for all, if, as mentioned, a quick-fix PK meal is needed at any time.

Please note, when following the plan below, that where there is advice to mix seeds with Coyo or Alpro yoghurt (see Other items), different people will have different tastes as to how 'thick' they would like this to be so experiment and find your preference.

Your weekly PK shop (by Craig)

The idea here is to keep things very simple and also to have foods that can be ordered online and delivered to your house so as to reduce energy expended on shopping expeditions. I have included seven breakfasts, seven lunches and seven suppers,and some snacks too – there is one snack per day in this list. Regarding drinks, do concentrate on water; limit coffee and tea to a maximum of three cups a day.

For ease of shopping, in Table 7.2 I have listed the items and how to search for them on Ocado; where items are not generally available from Ocado, I have included Amazon alternatives. Of course, other major supermarkets will also be able to provide most of what is needed in a 'one stop shop'. Once you have done one or two shops, things will become much easier.

If you look elsewhere, always look at the labels which detail the carbohydrate content of foods; these are very helpful. The carbohydrate values given on labels are normally total carbs which include all starches, sugars and fibre. I prefer to use net carbs (sugars and starches, with fibre excluded) on the grounds that fibre does not spike blood sugar but is fermented into short chain fatty acids. Linseed is a good example – it is low-carb because, although 100 grams contains 29 grams of total carb, 27 grams is fibre and so just 2 grams is starch and sugar. Please see the detailed explanatory note regarding food labelling in Chapter 2 (page 19).

You will need to tailor these suggestions to you personally so that you get into and remain in ketosis – do not take these suggested meals as guarantors of ketosis.

I have presented the shopping list in two ways:

1. By meal. This list has been compiled like this so that you can see what a daily meal plan might look like by choosing one breakfast, one lunch, one supper and a snack. There is also an 'Other items' list.
2. In one combined list, showing you what the total buy will be. This list has been compiled like this so that it is easy to follow and can be used by a carer to shop for you or by yourself or family member to order the items online. As I have said, I have included the search details for each item on Ocado and where Ocado does not (generally) stock items, I have included Amazon alternatives.

1. Shopping list by meals for one week (the seven-day meal plan)

Breakfasts for one week
- 3 x 'natural' Cocos yoghurt (125 g)
- 2 x vanilla Cocos yoghurt (125 g)
- 1 x Alpro vanilla yoghurt (500 g – to cover two breakfasts with a bit left over)

Lunches for one week

Seven starters:

- Two avocados (say, 200 g) with mayonnaise
- Large dollop mayonnaise
- Salami (just one 'stick')
- Celery stick and paté – celery (350 g - should last two meals; Farmhouse pork paté (100 g in two servings of 50 g – lasts two meals)
- Cucumber and tomato – cucumber (should last two meals); tomatoes (six-pack – should last two meals)
- Sauerkraut (350 g – should last three meals)
- Carrot and coconut soup (400 g)

Seven mains:

- Tinned ham (200 g – may have to make this last for two meals; 125 g would be ideal)
- Corned beef (200 g – may have to make this last for two meals; 125 g would be ideal)
- Tinned mackerel – in tomato sauce (125 g)
- Tinned tuna (160 g)
- Tinned sardines in spicy tomato (120 g)
- Quorn with mozzarella and pesto sauce(lasts two meals – see Table 7.2)
- Washed salad
- (**Occasional** coconut paleo wraps)

Seven puddings:

- Cocos natural yoghurt (125 g)
- Cocos vanilla yoghurt (125 g)
- Cocos mixed berry yoghurt (125 g)
- 50 g blueberries from freezer with dollop of coconut cream
- 50 g raspberries from freezer with dollop of coconut cream
- 50 g gooseberries from freezer with dollop of coconut cream
- 50 g strawberries from freezer with dollop of coconut cream

Suppers for one week
- Same starter, main and pudding suggestions as for Lunches – mix and match.

Snacks
- 2 x snacks - Black Country No Nonsense Pork Scratchings one bag – twice a week
- 2 x snacks - one bar Green and Black's 85% dark chocolate – half a bar counts as one snack – twice a week.
- 1 snack – one scoop of macadamia nut butter (or hazelnut nut butter)
- 1 snack olives - snack on say 30 g
- 1 snack – biltong - snack on say 25 g

Other items
- Chia seeds – say 50 g to add to yoghurts to taste, as and when
- Linseed – say 50 g to add to yoghurts to taste, as and when (lasts longer than one week)
- Coconut milk – to fill up on if you are still hungry at night (400 ml should last about one week; I prefer Grace Coconut Milk)
- Coconut cream – for use with berries as a pudding (200 g should last about a week)

Herbal teas/coffee
In addition, up to three cups per day. Select from:
www.tealyra.co.uk/loose-tea-uk/herbal-teas-uk/

2. Complete shopping list in one combined list for one week

The list in Table 7.2 covers all the food items needed for all the meals listed above for one week. Some of these items will last longer than one week; go by the advice above as to how much to eat.

Table 7.2: What foods to buy for one week and how to order them online

Shopping item	Go to Ocado and search for	If not on Ocado go to Amazon and search for:
5 x 'natural' Cocos yoghurt (125 g)	'Cocos Natural Yoghurt' and select size	
4 x Cocos vanilla yoghurt (125 g)	'Cocos Vanilla Yoghurt' and select size	
2 x Cocos mixed berry yoghurt (125 g)	'Cocos Mixed Berry Yoghurt' and select size	
1 x Alpro vanilla yoghurt 500 g	'Alpro Vanilla Yoghurt' and select size	
4 x avocados (100 g each)	'Avocados' and select size	
Mayonnaise	'Mayonnaise' and choose to your liking – 'Delouis' looks good	
Pack of six Serious Pig snacking salami	'Salami snacking' and choose your own if no 'Serious Pig' available – 'Rutland Charcuterie' looks good	'Serious Pig Classic Snacking Salami (pack of six)'
350 g celery	'Celery sticks 350 g'	
100 g Farmhouse Pork Pate	'Waitrose Farmhouse Pork Pate 100 g'	
One cucumber	'Cucumber' and select size – 'full wholefood organic' or 'Waitrose'	
Pack of six tomatoes	'6 tomatoes' – 'essential Waitrose' or 'Ocado'	
350 g pot organic sauerkraut	'Organic sauerkraut 350 g'	
Carrot and coconut soup 400 g	'Carrot and coconut soup'	
2 x 200 g tinned ham	'Tinned ham' and select size	
2 x 200 g corned beef	'Corned beef' and select size	

Shopping item	Go to Ocado and search for	If not on Ocado go to Amazon and search for:
2 x 125 mg tinned mackerel in tomato sauce	'Tinned mackerel, tomato' and select size	
Pack of 4 X 160 g tinned tuna	'Tinned tuna' and select size	
2 x 120 g tinned sardines in spicy tomato	'Tinned sardines, spicy' and select size	
2 wraps (240 g) Quorn – with mozzarella and pesto sauce	'Quorn mozzarella & Pesto escalopes 240 g'	
2 x washed salad in a bag	'Salad bag' and choose to your taste	
Pack of 14 paleo coconut wraps	No equivalent – expensive – Amazon purchase should last weeks	Or go to ukiherb.com and search for Julian Bakery Organic Paleo Wraps, 7 wraps, 7.7 oz (224 g)
150 g blueberries	'Blueberries' and select size	
150 g raspberries	'Raspberries' and select size	
200 g gooseberries	'Gooseberries' – these are 'British Cooking Gooseberries' – not always in stock – see opposite	Waitrose online stocks 'Cooks' Ingredients Gooseberries' and Sainsbury's online stock '400 g Gooseberries'
227 g strawberries	'Strawberries' and select size	
Black Country No Nonsense Pork Scratchings	'Pork crackling' and select your own if no 'Black Country' – 'Awfully Posh' crackling looks good	'Black Country No Nonsense Pork Scratchings (24 bags)'
Green and Black's 85% dark chocolate	'Green and Black's 85%' – one bar per week	
Macadamia nut butter	'Macadamia nut butter'	
Pot olives	'Olives' and choose to taste	
Biltong	'Biltong' and choose to taste	

Chia seeds	'Chia seeds' and choose to taste	
Linseed	'Linseed' and choose to taste	
Coconut milk	'400 ml coconut milk' and choose to taste	'Grace Coconut Milk'. You can order 12 x 1 litre cartons in one go.
Coconut cream	'Biona creamed coconut 200 g'	

I have eaten this diet for six weeks and I can confirm that:
- It got me into ketosis
- It kept me in ketosis
- I did get very bored of it by the fifth week
- I lost quite a lot of weight
- It wasn't too expensive.

So, this meal plan does exactly what it says on the tin! Craig.

Chapter 8

The PK bakery

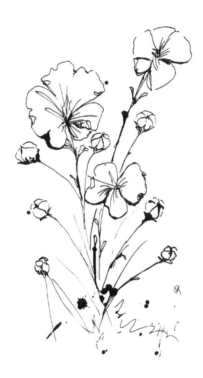

The single biggest reason for lapsing on the PK diet is the absence of bread. To secure the diet for life you must first make PK bread. I rose early for six months to experiment and so developed the recipe below. This is quick, easy and works reliably well. If you have any friends or family offering to help you, then top of the list must be: 'Please make my daily bread!'

> *Give us this day our daily bread.*
> The Lord's Prayer,* Matthew 6:9–13, English Standard Version, *The Bible*

PK bread consists of just linseed,† Sunshine salt and water. Americans, and others, may be more familiar with linseed being referred to as flax or flaxseed or common flax. There is technically a subtle difference - flax is grown as a fibre plant that is used for linen while linseed is grown for its seed. The flax plant is taller than linseed and is pulled by hand or nowadays by machine.

How to make PK buns or loaf in minutes

Please forgive the tiresome detail, but you must succeed with your first batch because then you will be encouraged to carry on. I can now put this recipe together in 5 minutes (proper minutes that is – not the 'and this is what I did earlier' TV version!). These days I always make buns as they cook more reliably well.

You can see me preparing this loaf on YouTube:

    Loaf: www.youtube.com/watch?v=bjwjUXxELb0

    Buns: www.youtube.com/watch?v=YKP13aWyw_8&list=PLJGxkcH41f8m9H-wHlDor56bpd4E44fynS&index=4

---

* **Footnote:** For me as a child this seemed the most important part of the Lord's prayer. I was amused to read of another child who discerned God's full name and address from listening to the Lord's prayer by hearing: 'Our Father Wichart in Heaven. Harold be thy name... lead us not into Thames Station'. A further account of a child witnessing Christian burial rites at the graveside listened to the priest signing off with '... unto the Father, unto the Son and unto the Holy Ghost' but heard '...and to the Father, and to the Son and into the hole he goes'. This still wakes me regularly at night bubbling and choking with laughter.

† Linseed's species is *Linum usitatissimum*, (Latin – 'the most useful linen') and it is a member of the genus Linum, being in the family Linaceae. The plant species is now seen only as a cultivated plant and it seems to have been domesticated only once from the (wild) species *Linum bienne* (pale flax). The evidence suggests that it was first domesticated for oil, rather than fibre.[1] *Linum usitatissimum* L. is one of eight main 'founder crops' domesticated in the Fertile Crescent about 11,000 years ago, although there is evidence of microscopic fibres from 30,000 years ago found in a cave in Georgia. It therefore originates in the crossover period between Palaeolithic and Neolithic eras.[2] (The Fertile Crescent is the region in the Middle East which curves, like a quarter-moon shape, from the Persian Gulf, through modern-day southern Iraq, Syria, Lebanon, Jordan, Israel and northern Egypt.)

Equipment needed:

Oven that gets to 220°C

Weighing scales

Measuring jug

Nutribullet (or similar effective grinding machine; do not attempt to do this with a pestle and
  mortar – I know – I have tried and failed)

Cup in which to weigh the linseed

Mixing bowl

Wooden spoon

A 500 g (or 1 lb in weight) baking tin (for loaf) or greased baking sheet (for buns)

Paper towels

Wire rack for cooling

Ingredients:

250 g linseeds (brown or golden)

1 tsp Sunshine salt

270 ml water

Dollop of coconut oil or lard

Actions	Notes
Take/weigh out 250 g whole linseed	You could purchase this in 250 g packs and that saves weighing it. Use golden grains to make a brown loaf; brown grains will be darker. Do not buy linseed that has already been ground because the grinding may not be fine enough; it may also have absorbed some water already and this may stop it sticking together and rising. If you purchase linseed in bulk, then you must weigh it really accurately in order to get the proportion of water spot on
Pour half the linseeds into the Nutribullet together with one rounded teaspoon of Sunshine salt Grind into a fine flour	Grind until the machine starts to groan and sweat with the effort. You need a really fine flour to make a good loaf. This takes about 30 seconds. The finer you can grind the flour the better it sticks together and the better the loaf. I have a small Nutribullet, so I do this in two batches or the blades 'hollow out' the mix so that half does not circulate and grind fully *and* you risk burning out the motor (and I have!)

Actions	Notes
Pour the ground flour into a mixing bowl	
Repeat the above with the second half of seeds and add to the mixing bowl	Whilst this is grinding, measure the water you need
Add seeds for flavour	My daughters complained the bread tasted fishy, so I now add a generous teaspoonful of caraway or cumin or fennel seeds If you wish to make a whole loaf, Sarah White advises a more reliable result by adding in ¾ tsp baking powder and 1½ dsp psyllium husks. Then bake at 200°C fan oven for 60-70 minutes (it's quite oven-specific)
Add in exactly 270 ml water (not a typo – 270 it is!) Chuck it all in at once; do not dribble it in. Stir it with a wooden spoon and keep stirring; it will thicken over the course of 30 seconds. Keep stirring until it becomes smooth and holds together in a lump	The amount of water is critical. When it comes to cooking, I am a natural chucker in of ingredients and hope for the best, but in this case, you must measure! Initially it will look as if you have added far too much water – keep stirring
Wait 15 minutes to allow the ground linseed to fully absorb the water	I often make up the dough the night before so I can have fresh bread for breakfast
Use your fingers to scoop up a dollop of coconut oil or lard to grease the baking tin	Your hands will be covered in fat which means you can pick up your dough without it sticking your hands
Use your hands to shape the dough until it has a smooth surface	Spend about 30 seconds doing this. Do not be tempted to knead or fold the loaf or you introduce layers of fat which stop it sticking to itself. This helps prevent the loaf cracking as it rises and cooks (although I have to say it does not matter two hoots if it does. It just looks more professional if it does not!)

For the loaf: Drop the mixture into the greased baking tin and bake inthe oven at at least 220°C (430°F) for 60 minutes	Set a timer or you will forget – I always do! I do not think the exact temperature is too critical, but it must be hot enough to turn the water in the loaf into steam because that is what raises it. I cook my bread on a wood-fired stove and the oven temperature is tricky to be precise with; That does not seem to matter so long as it is really hot. Indeed, I like the flavour of a slightly scorched crust
For the buns: Mould the dough into the shape of a rolling pin, then use a sharp knife to cut 12 discs. Place these onto a greased baking tray and cook in the oven at 220°C (430°F) for 40 minutes	Ditto above. These buns cook reliably well. Yes, you can make a whole loaf but so many have had disasters either with a soggy middle or a bucket-handle hole in the top of the loaf

Taste

At my first writing of this chapter I stated 'Do not expect this bread to taste and perform exactly like a conventional wheat-based loaf'. However, my PK bread recipe has evolved so much in the six months of experimentation that many of my greatest critics (one of whom is me!) have been won over. The resultant loaf, made with golden linseed, looks exactly like a small brown Hovis.[‡]

Even if the loaf does not initially taste good to you, keep at it. Taste is acquired. A dear friend and colleague – namely the late Dr Alan Franklin, consultant paediatrician at Chelmsford – ran a trial with his allergic children. They, too, had to avoid grains and dairy. With their agreement, Dr Franklin's patients ate a portion of their least favourite food daily. These included foods that kids often dislike, such as Brussels sprouts,[§]

[‡] **Footnote:** The name Hovis was coined in 1890 by London student Herbert Grime in a national competition set by S. Fitton & Sons Ltd to find a trading name for their patent flour which was rich in wheat germ. Grime won £25 when he coined the word from the Latin phrase *hominis vis* – 'the strength of man'. The company became the Hovis Bread Flour Company Limited in 1898.

[§] **Historical note:** Brussels sprouts seem to have had a mysterious history. Some sources indicate that they were eaten in classical times, but the evidence is not conclusive. English food writer Jane Grigson states that they are first mentioned in the city of Brussels market regulations in 1213, thus giving rise to their name. Mention of Brussels sprouts certainly appears about 200 years later on the menus of Burgundian wedding feasts held at the court of Lille.

mushrooms and avocado pears. No child had to eat the food more than 14 times (i.e. for two weeks) before coming to like it.

We are not born with taste preferences; we acquire them. Primitive man, pottering through the jungle, would have tried new foods with great suspicion and reluctance. However, if he was not poisoned, but rather nourished by that food, then he would eat more and more of it and eventually would come to like it. By way of association of sensation, taste and satiety, he would progress to actively seeking out that food. In the long term he would farm and harvest such.

The above scenario reflects my personal journey with linseed bread. I initially viewed my dark brown brick with distaste and suspicion. I forced it down out of a sense of loyalty to the diet. However, as I have perfected the above recipe I have come to look forward to and love it. It has character, texture and taste. It forms part of every breakfast and supper. My breakfast invariably has PK fried bread i.e. linseed bread fried in coconut oil or lard. My suppers often start with PK toast.

PK bread options

Many friends have come up with some great PK bakery ideas and I am grateful to all of them. Here they are – enjoy! I present them as they were sent to me – no standard layout for recipes here. Note they all have a higher carbohydrate content than the original above so do check you are staying in ketosis. Table 8.1 shows how different seed and nut flours compare with linseed for fibre and carb content – all are higher in carbs.

Table 8.1: Comparative fibre and carb contents of seed and nut flours

Seed or nut	Fibre % USDA figures	Carb% USDA figures	Notes
Linseed	27	2	The best PK seed 22% omega 3 oil (the best source of omega 3 for vegetarians)
Chia	34	8	High-fibre, so great for the lower fermenting gut (see Chapter 3). 18% omega 3 oil

Pumpkin	1	6	49% fat 26% omega 6 oil
Sunflower	9	11	30% omega 6
Sesame	12	11	20% omega 6
Almond flour	11	4	
Coconut flour	39	17	Very high in fibre, but high-carb so use sparingly. It absorbs large amounts of fluid

So beware, the recipes below all have a higher carbohydrate content than the basic PK loaf. The principles of baking are as above. I start with four from naturopath and naturopathic bodyworker Mim Elkan.

Seed loaf

- 250 ml water
- 6 g (I rounded tsp) sea salt

Grind:
- 80 g sunflower seeds
- 80 g pumpkin seeds
- 40 g sesame seeds
- 40 g chia seeds
- 60 g whole linseed

Leave whole:
- 20 g sunflower seeds
- 20 g pumpkin seeds

Yussuf's loaf

This is Mim's favourite – high-sesame; low-linseed.

- 150 ml water
- 6 g (1 rounded tsp) sea salt

Grind:
- 120 g sunflower seeds
- 90 g pumpkin seeds
- 70 g sesame seeds
- 30 g chia seeds
- 20 g whole linseed (dark or golden linseed or a mix)

Leave whole:
- 20 g sunflower seeds
- 20 g pumpkin seeds

High-sunflower seed; low-linseed; no chia seed; drier loaf

- 150 ml water
- 6 g (1 rounded tsp) sea salt

To grind:
- 120 g sunflower seeds
- 80 g pumpkin seeds
- 40 g sesame seeds
- 60 g whole linseed

Leave whole:
- 20 g sunflower seeds
- 20 g pumpkin seeds

I like this one!

- 200 ml water
- 6 g (1 rounded tsp) sea salt

Grind:
- 100 g sunflower seeds
- 80 g pumpkin seeds
- 40 g sesame seeds
- 20 g chia seeds
- 60 g whole linseed

Leave whole:
- 20 g sunflower seeds
- 20 g pumpkin seeds

Optional extras

- Some walnuts, pecans or other nuts – ground and/or in small pieces
- Herbs and spices: e.g. cumin seed, caraway seed, coriander seed, smoked paprika, cinnamon, nutmeg
- 5 g (1 level tsp) psyllium husk
- 20 g hemp seeds
- ½ tsp baking powder

Philippa Sherwood's linseed, turmeric and cauliflower bread

This is a very quick and easy, tasty, versatile starch-free, gluten-free, wheat-free bread. It will store in the fridge for up to five days.

330 g (2 cups) cauliflower
3 eggs or 4 egg whites
100 g ground linseed
2-3 tsp turmeric, ground

Pinch freshly ground black pepper
2 tsp baking powder – optional
½ tsp salt or less

1. Grate the cauliflower. However, I use a Russell Hobbs Mini mincer which I've had for ages, but similar online is RH 2032056 desire, 300w. It breaks the cauliflower down to very small pieces, although it doesn't matter if it is coarse or broken down fairly fine.
2. Weigh the ground linseed into a bowl and add the other dry ingredients, including the turmeric, and mix thoroughly.
3. Beat the eggs and add to the mix. Mix thoroughly.
4. Tip the 'bread' mix into a large baking tray and spread out thinly.
5. Place in 175°C oven and cook until golden brown. This should take about 25 minutes but depends on thickness and individual oven.
6. Cool and cut into slices.

Note: What works for me

I add a little more turmeric than they say.

I spread on two baking sheets – one thinly, one thickly, and bake. The thick ones I bake for longer. I then freeze them and use when needed – they thaw very quickly, or I put them under the grill lightly or fry.

Some of the thin ones, when cooked, I cut and then bake again very slowly in a very low oven (100/150°C) for a while, so they become crispy. I like the change of texture – they're more like a hard biscuit. I spread sesame seed paste on them and add crushed fresh fruit as a 'jam' for tea.

Christina Macleod's flaxseed crackers

The following is enough for 10 crackers.
Preparation time 5 minutes (easy and delicious)
Cooking time 25 minutes in a cooker

2 level tbsp flaxseeds/linseeds (I grind these in the coffee grinder)
30 ml or 2 tbsp water approx
I tsp favourite herbs

1. Mix everything together and rest for 2-3 minutes.
2. Place the meal on baking paper, then place another sheet on top and press or roll out between the sheets of paper until between 2 and 3 mm.
3. Deeply score the rolled mixture into cracker-sized rectangles. This will ensure that they break into evenly sized crackers; then put top sheet back.
4. Cook in a preheated oven at 180°C/gas 5-6 for 2 to 30 minutes until dry but not burnt, or microwave for 2.5 minutes or until the meal is hard.
5. Stand for a couple of minutes until the biscuits are cool to the touch.
6. Crack apart and store in an airtight container.

Carolyn Chesshire's linseed biscuits

I cup ground linseed
Sunshine salt to taste
4 tbsp sesame/sunflower/pumpkin seeds (whichever/whatever mixture; suggest if sunflower/
  pumpkin you grind them up a bit)
2 tbsp dried thyme/sage/mix herbs/dried chilli/coriander powder/cumin seeds/powder…
  whatever you like
½ cup cold water

1. Mix the dry ingredients together in a bowl and add the water, then mix to a dough.
2. Sometimes I add 2 tsp of finely chopped onion and 1 tsp crushed garlic – the flavourings are whatever you want them to be.
3. Tip onto a sheet of baking parchment, top with another sheet of baking parchment and flatten with your hand, then roll out.
4. Lightly score the flattened mix in order to break into biscuits when cooked.
5. Slide the baking parchment onto a baking sheet and chuck in a hot oven for as long as the biscuits cook and turn lightly brown. I just watch them as they go along and break off/remove cooked ones as they become ready…. You'll soon get the idea. They are delicious!

Dee Marshall's paleo chocolate cake

For feast days only.

I cup ground almonds
½ cup smooth almond butter
3 large eggs, separated
3 tbsp maple syrup
½ cup unsweetened stewed apple
¼ cup organic raw cacao powder
I tsp baking soda
I tsp vanilla extract
1/8 tsp salt

1. Preheat the oven to 180°C.
2. Line a 20-cm/8-inch cake tin with greaseproof paper.
3. Whisk the egg whites until firm.
4. Whisk the egg yolks separately.
5. Add all the ingredients except the egg whites to a mixing bowl and mix well with an electric whisk or a wooden spoon.
6. Fold in the egg whites carefully to keep as much air in as possible for a lighter texture.
7. Pour the mixture into the cake tin.
8. Bake for 25-27 minutes until a cocktail stick comes out clean.
9. Cool completely before taking out of the tin.
10. When completely cool, top with melted unsweetened dark chocolate, or coconut cream and melted chocolate mixed: Melt 1½-2 x 100 g bars of dark chocolate in the microwave for about a minute, or in a bowl over hot water. Heat up the cream only from the top of a tin of coconut milk and pour into the melted chocolate. Cool slightly before using it to ice the cake.

Jason O'Sullivan's PK scones

Make these in the same way as the PK buns but add to the dry mixture:

- Raisins
- Cinnamon
- Goji berries
- Nutmeg (enough to smell/be visible)

Then add the water.
Bake in a preheated oven at 200-220°C or less for approximately 20 minutes.

Moira Creak's beetroot flaxseed crackers

These are delicious with hummus, guacamole or a creamy vegan cheese dip. The following ingredients will make 30 crackers.

100 g ground almonds or sunflower seeds
60 g grated raw beetroot
90 g whole flaxseeds
1 tsp garlic powder or finely grated fresh garlic
1 tbsp herbs or spices, such as fennel seeds, *herbes de Provence* or fresh or dried thyme or
    rosemary
½ tsp sea salt

1. Preheat the oven to fan 180°C/Gas mark 6, if using.
2. In a large bowl, combine all the ingredients with your hands to make a dough, but don't overmix or it will become too moist.
3. Bring the dough together into a ball and roll it between two sheets of baking parchment to a 3 mm thickness. When rolling out, try and roll into a neat rectangle with straight edges as this will make it easier to snap off good-sized, evenly baked crackers.
4. Keeping the top layer of baking parchment in place, gently mark the dough through the paper into 5-cm squares with the back of a knife, without breaking the

paper. Carefully peel back the top piece of baking paper.

5. Transfer the bottom layer, with the scored cracker dough, directly onto the oven shelf, rack or dehydrator shelf. (If using a dehydrator, dehydrate at 45°C for 8 hours until crisp.)

6. Bake in the oven for 12 minutes, then check the crackers. The ones on the outside will be nicely toasted and golden, so snap these off and put to one side (they will crisp up as they cool). Return the rest of the crackers to the oven for a few more minutes, until also crisp and toasted.

7. Leave the crackers to cool on a wire rack for 20 minutes, then finish snapping them and enjoy alone or serve with dips. They will keep for one week in a sealed container in the fridge.

Sarah's pizza

For the dough mix:

75 g golden flaxseeds, ground
50 ml water
125 g vegan 'mozzarella', coarsely grated
100 g ground almonds
3 eggs
1 tsp baking powder
1 tsp Sunshine salt

1. Preheat the oven to 200°C/180°C fan/Gas 6.
2. Line a baking tray with baking parchment and brush with oil.
3. Mix the dough ingredients together in a large bowl until thoroughly combined or give them a quick whizz in a food processor. The flaxseed will absorb the moisture and thicken it in minutes.
4. Use one hand to gather the dough into a ball, leaving the bowl clean.
5. Wet your hands and flatten the dough into an oval shape on the baking tray to a thickness of just over 1 cm all over.
6. Cook for 15 to 20 minutes or until golden-brown.
7. Then add whatever pizza topping you fancy and cook for a bit longer:

Tomato, onion, chopped leeks, peppers (whatever is in the garden, even lettuce and salad leaves work well)
Smoked fish, salami chunks, vegan cheese
Tinned anchovies, prawns
Salt, pepper, tomato paste, pesto, chilli powder

Keto pastry for quiche

½ cup almond flour
½ cup coconut flour
2 tbsp psyllium husk powder
2 tbsp coconut oil
2 large eggs
5 tbsp ice-cold water
¼ tsp Sunshine salt

1. Mix together the dry ingredients in a bowl.
2. Scramble the eggs in a small bowl or measuring cup and let them sit for a moment.
3. Add the coconut oil to the dry ingredients and work it into the flours. You should end up with a sandy consistency.
4. Add the beaten eggs to the bowl and mix in well.
5. Add ice-cold water until you reach a consistency where you can work with the dough – it looks a bit sandy as you're mixing, but as you use your hands, it should stick together.
6. Knead the dough into a ball and let it sit for 5 minutes; the coconut flour and psyllium absorb the water and this hold it all together.
7. Form the ball of dough into a square and cut out 4-5 sections.
8. Use as you would pastry – press into a tart dish and par-cook the dough for 12-15 minutes at 350°F.
9. Fill it with whatever you'd like – eggs, onion, tomato, bacon, salami, vegan cheese….
10. Cook for another 20-30 minutes with the filling in place.

Carolyn Chesshire's keto pancakes

I cup almond flour
I tbsp coconut flour
3 eggs
$^1/_3$ cup coconut milk
Lemon juice to taste

1. Mix the almond flour with the coconut flour.
2. Mix in the eggs with the coconut milk; this gives you a batter which you can cook and flip.
3. Flavour with lemon juice, if you like.

Chapter 9

The PK dairy

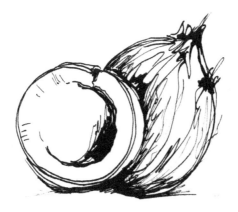

Giving up dairy products was, for me, like a bereavement. I so loved butter, cheese and cream! In the early 1980s the only alternative was a thin grey liquid called soya milk. Now we have great alternatives largely because coconut milk and palm oil have the almost identical medium-chain fats to dairy products. These fats impart a similar smooth texture which means that we can make excellent dairy alternatives and I no longer feel deprived.

Table 9.1: No-cook quickly-prepared alternatives to dairy

	PK options	Notes
PK milk	Soya milk, coconut milk and other such nut milks	Choose those that are non-GM and free from sweeteners
PK single cream	Grace coconut milk at room temperature	Comprised solely of coconut milk and water; fabulous creamy texture; an absolute essential for the PK diet. Note the carton form is far superior to the tinned form – dunno why
PK double cream	Grace coconut milk from the fridge	Ditto
PK yoghurt	Cocos	Choose the plain yoghurt as the flavoured varieties have added fruit or sugar. See recipe below
PK butter	Vegan block 'Naturli' is my favourite	Do not use this for cooking as it contains some unsaturated oils
PK cheese	The vegan cheeses are not quite the same as dairy cheeses but make a very acceptable substitute. My favourites are the Bute Island 'sheeses' www.buteisland.com	A bit pricey so I use them sparingly; they do contain yeast, so yeast allergics beware
PK ice cream	An ultra-quick version is simply to pour Grace coconut milk over frozen berries and put in the deep freeze for a few minutes	This is my staple pudding because it is so quick and easy
PK chocolate	85-100% dark chocolate	A bar of this lasts me several days. This tells me I am not addicted to it. Most people are addicted to the sugar and dairy content of chocolate – I know this from my own experience as a bar of 'normal' less than 85% coco-solids chocolate I cannot ignore

Table 9.2: Dairy-substitutes that need time, energy and inclination

	Ingredients	Actions
PK super-thick double-cream	Grace coconut milk 80% Coconut oil 20% ½ tsp lecithin per 500 ml	Pour the coconut milk and lecithin into the Nutribullet or equivalent. Warm up the oil so it pours and add to the milk. Whizz up for a few seconds. Put in the fridge and it sets to double-cream consistency
PK clotted cream	As above but use Grace coconut milk 60% and coconut oil 40%	As above
PK yoghurt	Grow kefir on soya or coconut milk as detailed in Chapter 18: Fermented foods Pour off excess whey Coconut oil 20% ½ tsp lecithin per 500 ml	Pour the soya or coconut milk kefir and lecithin into the Nutribullet or equivalent. Warm up the oil so it pours and add to the milk. Whizz up for a few seconds. Put in the fridge and it sets to double-cream consistency
PK ice cream – quick version	Cup of Grace coconut milk ¼ tsp lecithin Frozen berries – not more than a handful or they clog up in the machine. Optional: Add gelatin to reduce ice crystals forming	Make this in small batches otherwise it freezes solid and will not mix. Pour coconut milk and lecithin into the Nutribullet (or equivalent). Add frozen berries and immediately whizz it all up before it freezes; it should turn into a slush. Pour into small container and freeze. If I want a large amount, I do this in several small batches; a film of coconut milk on the inside helps to prevent it setting solid in the Nutribullet. I have done it wrong lots of time by being greedy and doing too big a batch at once. You will too! But. again, as Marcel Proust said, 'We must discover it for ourselves'
PK ice cream – long version	Ingredients as above, but…	…sieve out the skins and pips and put the slush into an ice cream maker. This stirs the mix constantly so preventing ice crystals forming and imparts that wonderful silky-smooth texture. I rarely make this because the above version is so quick, so easy and so good, with minimal washing up *and* contains all the goodness of the berry skins. I told you I was lazy!

	Ingredients	Actions
PK coconut chocolate	1 x whole 460-g pot of coconut oil
For mild chocolate add the same volume of pure cocoa powder (or 1 x 125 g pot of Greens and Blacks cocoa powder).
For dark chocolate add twice the amount – i.e. 2 x 125 pots of Green and Blacks.
(You can of course make this using pure cocoa butter, but this is rather expensive)	Pour the coconut oil into a pan and warm.
Add the pure cocoa powder/Greens and Blacks cocoa powder.
Mix together.
Pour into ice cube containers and put in the deep freeze.
Eat this PK chocolate direct from the deep freeze. It melts in the mouth just like chocolate. Coconut oil has a lower melting point than chocolate fat – it will run off the table if served at room temperature

Chapter 10

PK breakfasts

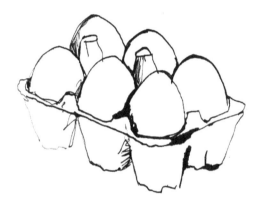

Remember, an army marches on its stomach.

Have a good breakfast men, for we dine in Hades!
King Leonidas' words to his soldiers before the Battle of Thermopylae, 480 BC*

Breakfast is the most important meal of the day, but also the one on which we least want to spend physical and mental energy. For this reason, most people have the same breakfast each day which they can make without thinking. This frees the active brain to organise the day ahead.

'When you wake up in the morning, Pooh,' said Piglet at last, 'what's the first thing you say to yourself?'
'What's for breakfast?' said Pooh. 'What do you say, Piglet?'
'I say, I wonder what's going to happen exciting today?' said Piglet.
Pooh nodded thoughtfully. 'It's the same thing,' he said.
Winnie the Pooh by A A Milne, 18 January 1882 – 31 January 1956

* Footnote: Hopefully things will not end the same way for us as it did for the Spartans, although they did achieve a kind of immortality... During the second Persian invasion of Greece (480 BC), King Leonidas of Sparta, with his 300 Spartans, and possibly up to 700 Thespians and some Helots and Thebans, took a tactical decision to block the only road pass that the Persians, led by Xerxes I, could take into Europe, near Thermopylae. According to Herodotus (see below), Xerxes led an army of over 1 million men, but modern scholars put this figure nearer to 150,000. The Spartans stood at the narrow pass of Thermopylae and held off the Persians for three days, but they and the Thespians all lost their lives. The Thebans surrendered. The three days that Leonidas had deliberately 'bought' gave the rest of the Greek city states the time they needed to collect their fleets, decide on a plan and decisively defeat the Persian fleet at Salamis. Xerxes could see that the Greeks were attempting to encircle his army and so he retreated from Europe, losing most of his men to starvation and disease. The following year the Greeks inflicted a final defeat on the Persians at Plataea. The '300' lost their lives in an heroic act of almost unbelievable courage. The Battle of Thermopylae has gone down in history as the 'Battle that saved Western Civilisation'. Had Leonidas not held that pass for those three days, then Greece and subsequently all European civilisation, most likely would have fallen to the Persians. The British novelist, playwright and poet, William Golding (1911 – 1993) wrote: 'A little of Leonidas lies in the fact that I can go where I like and write what I like. He contributed to setting us free.' Interested readers should see https://en.wikipedia.org/wiki/Battle_of_Thermopylae or listen to the wonderful Melvyn Bragg and experts discuss this battle on the episode 'Thermopylae' of BBC Radio 4's *In Our Time* at www.bbc.co.uk/programmes/p004y278. *Very* interested readers should read Herodotus's account (available at: https://penelope.uchicago.edu/Thayer/E/Roman/Texts/Herodotus/7d*.html).
Herodotus (c.484 BC – c.425 BC) was an Ancient Greek writer, geographer and historian who is best known for his *Histories* (available in their entirety at https://files.romanroadsstatic.com/materials/herodotus.pdf), and is therefore known as the 'Father of History'.

Table 10.1: Cooked breakfast with minimal time and effort

Cooked breakfast	Using the oven with an oven tray with a metal rack above	Notes
Meat: bacon, burgers, belly pork, sausage, black pudding etc	Place on top of the wire rack with strips of leaf fat or dripping	This leaves delicious crunchy scratchings as the fat runs away
PK bread, mushrooms, leftover green vegetables, onions, tomato, pepper or whatever	Under the rack place your PK bread and PK vegetables	The fat runs from upstairs to downstairs so the PK bread and vegetables soak it up and cook
	Put it all in the oven at 200°C. Set the timer for 15 minutes; this allows you to get on with other jobs but not burn your breakfast	
	When the timer goes off, crack an egg or two into the downstairs veggie tray - the heat of the tray will cook it. Tip onto plate and tuck in	Do not wash out the oven tray. Leave any fat in it for the next day. Indeed, it is my opinion that fat left like this at room temperature for 24 hours is far safer than washing up and risking traces of washing up liquid; detergent is highly toxic to the body. I still use Mother's cast iron pan – it has not been washed up for 58 years to my knowledge and probably longer

If you cannot face a *full* cooked breakfast, then see the suggestions below. However, my experience is that, given enough practice, not only can you, but it becomes a highly desirable part of the day.

The suggestions that follow sometimes require (some) cooking and sometimes little or none, but they are all designed to be less 'heavy' on the stomach, until you are ready for the Full Monty,[†] as above.

[†] **Historical note:** The origins of the phrase the 'full monty' are not known for certain, but, interestingly, one possibility is the enormous breakfasts eaten by Field Marshall Montgomery. It is said that the phrase was taken up after the War, presumably by ex-servicemen, as a name for the traditional English breakfast of bacon, eggs, fried bread, tomato, mushrooms, toast and cup of tea.

PK porridge

I cup ground linseeds
4 cups Grace coconut milk

1. Cook the linseed and coconut milk together in a pan for 30-60 seconds until the mixture thickens.
2. Serve.
3. You can add in berries and/or cinnamon.

PK muesli

I cup ground linseeds
4 cups Grace coconut milk
I dollop coconut or soya yoghurt
Nuts, seeds and/or berries, to taste

1. Combine the ground linseeds and coconut milk.
2. Allow to stand for a few minutes for the linseed to absorb the coconut milk.
3. Add the coconut or soya yoghurt.
4. Add in the nuts etc – see Appendix 3 for suggestions and carb content.

PK toast

PK buns or toast (toasted PK bread) with:

PK butter – Vegan block *Naturli* (see Chapter 9)
2-3 boiled eggs (now that I have ducks, this has become a regular breakfast)
smoked fish, tinned fish, tinned cod's roe
paté or rillette
vegan cheese and tomato
Cocos yoghurt

Also see Michelle McCullagh's Liver Pancakes in Chapter 22: The carnivore diet.

Smoothies

The key to a ketogenic smoothie is to ensure high fat and fibre content, but low sugar and starch. The oily basis of the smoothie should be:

avocado
coconut oil, or indeed
any nut, seed or vegetable oil
PLUS
1 tsp lecithin – this ensures the oil and water components are well blended to afford a
    wonderful silky-smooth texture
Possibly add soya or coconut yoghurt (Cocos) or Grace coconut milk
Choose salad and veg ad lib from Appendix 3: Green list (page 197), and more sparingly others
    from the amber list (page 198).

Craig's[‡] all-time favourite breakfasts

Asparagus cooked in PK butter topped with ham and PK cheese.
Scrambled eggs with PK butter and smoked salmon.

Also see:
    Michelle McCullagh's Liver pancakes in Chapter 22
    The 'no preparation' breakfasts in Chapter 7.

Shakespeare provides us with only one breakfast recipe:

> *Eight wild boars roasted whole at breakfast, but twelve persons there.*
>   *Antony and Cleopatra* Act 2, Scene 1, William Shakespeare,
>   26 April 1564 (baptised) – 23 April 1616

[‡] **Footnote:** During his days trying to regulate the City, in the early 1990s, Craig was often taken to what the traders called 'the Canteen' (actually the Savoy Grill), presumably to butter him up. It never worked, but Craig did get a taste for the scrambled eggs and smoked salmon, and even achieved that 'fame' of being able to enter the Savoy Grill and say to the waiter, 'My usual please, and he's paying!'

Chapter 11

PK starters

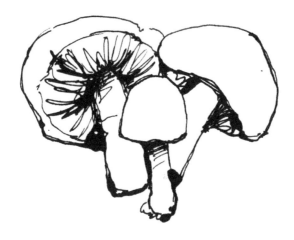

The origin of the 'starter' goes back a long way. Wealthy Romans generally had two main courses and before these courses they were served with small amounts of fish, vegetables, olives and even stuffed dormice – the usual stuffing was minced pork, pepper and pine kernels. These starters were known, most often, as *gustatio*.

> *Please, sir, I want some more.*
> Oliver, *Oliver Twist*, Charles Dickens, 7 February 1812 – 9 June 1870

Of course, tuck in!

Dr Sarah Myhill (1958 - 2058, horse falls permitting)

The following ideas are listed here in order of ease – i.e. those that require little time, energy or inclination come first:

- Bowl of sauerkraut – see Chapter 18: Fermented foods.
- PK bread or PK toast:
  - Dipped in oils e.g. olive, hemp or rape seed oil (another favourite but makes a mess of my shirt as I throw oil down the front of it – neither I nor the shirt mind too much but the person sitting opposite may! The dog is awfully pleased…)
  - With dripping and generous pinch of Sunshine salt and pepper
  - With palm oil or coconut oil
  - Dipped in PK yoghurt with garlic
  - With PK cheese and tomato.
- Anchovies (my favourite) – the oil in anchovies is particularly desirable to the brain being rich in the omega 3 fatty acid, EPA (eicosapentaenoic acid)
- Smoked fish, tinned cod's roe , sardines, crab, shellfish (mussels, cockles, whelks and winkles) with samphire
- Pate – there are many excellent patés which can be purchased or see below for PK recipe
- Rillette and brawn (see Chapter 22)
- Salami
- Sundried tomatoes
- Herb spreads e.g. pesto
- Olive paté
- Guacamole – blend avocado and tomato with herbs and French dressing
- Asparagus, globe artichokes with French dressing
- Large salad or coleslaw with French dressing or mayonnaise (see Chapter 13)
- Avocado.

Chapter 11

PK soup

If you are a particular lover of soup, you may consider purchasing a soup maker.* These are brilliant – you simply chuck in all the ingredients and it chops, cooks and blends so that you have a fabulous soup 20 minutes later.

Bone broth (see Chapter 22)
Vegetables – whatever is in the garden, pantry, deep freeze or delivered veggie box; eat
    seasonally
Herbs and spices that you like (for me this is garlic, black pepper, ginger, whatever is in the
    garden)

1. Chuck in your chosen ingredients.
2. Once the soup is cooked and cooled a little, stir in a large dollop of coconut milk
   (or other oil e.g. oil or hemp) if you wish for a creamier result.

PK gazpacho†

Salad vegetables including cucumber, tomatoes, lettuce, fennel, peppers, onions
French dressing

1. In the Nutribullet blend the salad veg.
2. Add a slug of French dressing.
3. Do not cook!
4. Eat with PK bread and PK garlic butter.

* **Note from Craig:** Sarah bought me a soup maker – it is so easy that even I can use it. There is virtually no effort required.

† **Historical note:** 'Gazpacho' goes back to the Romans. Roman legionaries used to carry dried bread, garlic and vinegar and any other pieces of salad and other vegetables that they could find, to make impromptu cold, raw soups during rest periods. The idea was taken up in southern Spain and then there was a merging of Moorish soups and the derived form of the Roman legionaries' 'soup'. This took place in the Andalusian area of Spain during the 8th Century AD. As to the name, one possible theory is that it derives from the Greek word for a collection box in church (γαζοφυλάκιον) where the congregation would contribute many different shaped coins, and even bread, to the church coffers; therefore, being a reference to the diversity of the contents of the soup.

Liver paté

Liver (pig, lamb, chicken, duck etc), as fresh as is possible
Fat for cooking
1 onion, raw, sliced
Sunshine salt
Pepper

1. Slice the liver and briefly fry it in an abundance of fat so the middle remains pink.
2. Tip the entire contents of the pan, fat and all, into the Nutribullet with the onion and seasoning.
3. Whizz up for a few seconds.
4. Transfer to a ceramic pot and keep in the fridge.

Carolyn's aubergine‡ dip

2 medium aubergines
2 tbsp extra-virgin olive oil
1 clove garlic, crushed
1 tbsp lemon juice (or your French dressing mix)
1 tbsp tahini
1 tbsp chopped mint
1 tbsp chopped parsley
½ tsp ground cumin

---

‡ **Historical note:** Originally aubergines come from India and Sri Lanka. The French term 'aubergine' derives from the historical city of Vergina (Βεργίνα) in Greece, where imports were probably first landed and is estimated to have reached the Greeks around 325 BC after the death of Alexander the Great in Babylon.

§ **Historical aside:** The name 'cracker' purportedly comes from a fateful day in 1801 in Massachusetts when Josiah Bent accidentally burned a batch of what we now call crackers. As the crackers burned, they made a crackling noise, and this inspired the name. Bent saw a good thing and by 1810, Bent's cracker business was successful and eventually was acquired by the National Biscuit Company (Nabisco). You can still buy crackers made by the company Bent's grandson founded, G.H. Bent Co. but these are distinctly not PK, unlike the delicious version opposite.

Topping:
I tbsp pomegranate seeds
a little olive oil

1. Preheat the oven to 200°C/180°C fan/Gas 6
2. Prick the aubergines with a fork, then cook whole on a baking tray for 45 minutes until the skins blister and the flesh is soft.
3. When cool, split the aubergines lengthways and scoop out the flesh.
4. Process (in the Nutribullet or equivalent) the flesh with the oil, garlic, lemon juice, tahini, mint, parsley and cumin to make a thick dip.
5. Season with black pepper.
6. Transfer to a serving dish.
7. Drizzle over the remaining olive oil and scatter the pomegranate seeds on top.
8. Serve with linseed crackers (see next).

Linseed crackers[§]

160 g golden or brown flaxseeds
80 g seeds – pumpkin, sunflower, sesame
Water to soak seeds
I tsp spice – cayenne, smoked paprika or other
½ sea salt

1. Put the flaxseeds in a bowl, pour over enough water to cover, and leave overnight.
2. Place the mixed seeds in a separate bowl, pour over enough water to cover and leave overnight.
3. Next morning, drain the flaxseeds and drain and rinse the mixed seeds.
4. Add the mixed seeds to the flaxseeds, which will have a jelly-like texture.
5. Add the salt and spice and transfer to a blender.
6. Pulse a few times to break up the seeds (but do not over-pulse – you want the seeds to be ground but still a little chunky).
7. Preheat the oven to 50°C/120°F.
8. Spread a very thin, even layer of the seed mix on a few waxed baking paper sheets.

9. Bake for approximately 6 hours, turning over halfway through to help the drying process.
10. Remove from the oven and allow to cool completely on the baking sheet.
11. Cut into squares with a knife or break into pieces.
12. The crackers can be stored in an airtight container for 2-4 weeks.

Variations:
- Seaweed and seed crackers – substitute 1 tbsp spirulina powder and 1 tbsp dried dulse flakes for the spice.
- Curry and seed crackers – substitute ½ tbsp curry powder and 1 tsp garlic powder for the spice.
- Sundried tomato and Italian herb crackers – Drain 12 sundried tomatoes packed in olive oil and pat dry; process in a food processor until smooth; substitute 1 tsp mixed Italian herbs, 1 tsp garlic powder and the blended sundried tomatoes for the spice.

Chapter 12

PK main courses
– stews and roasts

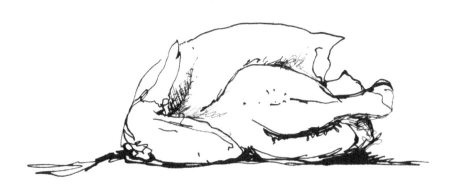

Stews

The formula for making good stews is the same regardless of the meat used – beef, pork, lamb, chicken, venison, pheasant, rabbit…. The cheaper and tougher the cut and the older the animal, the more flavour it has – neck or breast, oxtail, shin. Mutton is tastier than lamb.

1. Cut the meat into lumps and roll it in linseed or coconut flour, with Sunshine salt,

pepper and spices. My favourites are cumin, coriander* and cardamon.

2. Then flash fry the floured meat in a frying pan with plenty of fat to impart another dimension of delicious flavour. Remember, do not fry with oils.

3. Lob the browned meat into a slow-cooker with tomatoes, onions, leeks, garlic, herbs, whatever you like. If you like spicy stews, add ginger or chilli.

4. Cover with bone broth (see page 42) – an essential element – or add any available bones and cover with water.

5. Slow cook for hours.

6. If you have overdone the liquid, either leave the lid off so water evaporates off or thicken with coconut flour.

7. At the last moment, stir in a handful of herbs, garlic or garam marsala (thank you Shideh – yours is the best – see page 146) to provide a bouquet.

8. To accompany stews, try cauliflower 'rice': grate a cauliflower head and fry in pig or beef fat.

Roasts

The joy of a roast is that it is so quick and easy. You just stick the meat in the oven. Meat for roasting is always expensive because it reflects the ease of cooking. Again, roasts are all cooked to a simple formula which is as shown in Table 12.1.

---

* **Literary aside:** The word 'coriander' derives from the Old French *coriandre*, which comes originally from the Greek κορίαννον *koriannon*, possibly derived from or related to κόρις *kóris* (a bed bug) and was given on account of its bed-bug-like smell. Both Sarah and I love the taste and smell.[1]

† **To quote:** 'Tis an ill cook that cannot lick his own fingers.' *Romeo and Juliet*, Act IV Scene 2, William Shakespeare, 26 April 1564 (baptised) – 23 April 1616.

Table 12.1: The rules of a good roast

Action	Tricks of the trade
Take a lump of meat - beef, pork, lamb, venison, chicken, duck, goose, pheasant	With pork dishes, cut off the skin together with a layer of fat. The skin I cook separately to make perfect crackling. If the skin is cooked on the joint you risk eating good crackling and dry meat, or perfect meat and soggy crackling. Why not have good crackling and perfect meat?
Place in a roasting tray and cover with lard	The flavour is in the fat – ideally use strips of peritoneal or leaf fat. This leaves delicious crispy scratchings on the top of the joint. I generally scoff these before they get to the table.[†]
Put a whole onion into the roasting tin	Leave the onion skin on: this imparts great flavour and browns the gravy. (Thank you, Rosemary, for that tip)
Put in a hot oven, say 220°C. Set the timer for 30 minutes	The cooks tell me this 'seals' the outside of the joint and stops flavour leaking out. I am not so sure this is correct but, hey ho – it works in practice
When the timer goes off, take the joint out of oven and baste with the fat which will have run off. Reduce the temperature to 180°C. Reset the timer – see opposite for timings…	The total cooking time should be about 20 minutes per lb (0.45 kg), but less per lb if it is a very large joint. With experience you will get a feel for this. A meat thermometer takes the guess work out. Stick it in the thickest part of the joint and generally a temperature of 74°C (165°F) means it is cooked. You will quickly work out if this is too much or too little for taste. I like my joints pink on the inside
When the timer goes off, remove the joint from oven and lift onto a carving dish. Cover it with grease proof paper and a towel. Allow it to 'rest' for 30 minutes	The meat continues to cook at this lower temperature without drying out so remains succulent
For the gravy: Turn your attention back to the roasting tin. Pick up the onion and squeeze the soft centre out. Chuck the outside of the onion into the bone broth pot. Add garlic to the tin. Add bone broth. Put on to the cooker and heat – mash the onion in and scrape the brown bits off the bottom. Stir. If necessary, thicken with coconut flour	The most gorgeous gravy results. Serve. Use PK bread to mop up the juices if there is not enough veg to do the job. Worse – I suggest my dining companions look away – tip the plate up and slurp excess gravy up direct. It makes an impolite noise but is another highlight of my meal. The dog looks on anxiously to make sure I do not lick the plate too…

Michelle's stuffing

For the turkey, chicken, duck or goose

1 squash
2 onions
Lard for frying
Sausage meat (same amount as squash flesh)
2 eggs
Herbs – sage, oregano
Garlic, chopped
Sunshine salt
Black pepper

1. Pop the squash in the oven at 170°C and bake until soft. Timing depends on the size and type of squash. Crown prince squash are marvellous.
2. Take the squash out of oven and leave to cool.
3. Once cooled, scoop out the pips (scatter these on a roasting tray with a sprinkling of Sunshine salt and pop back in the oven to make a crispy snack).
4. Chop up the onions and fry up in lard until soft and juicy. Leave to cool.
5. Scoop a double handful of squash flesh into a large bowl, add the sausage meat, onions, eggs, herbs, garlic and generous salt and pepper.
6. Mix together and stuff it up the bird – voila, it is marvellous!

Shepherd's pie

Instead of potato use swede or squash

Pastry topping

200 g plain soya yoghurt
200 g smooth almond butter
2 eggs
1 tbsp lemon juice
¼ tsp sea salt
Pine nuts (optional)

1. Combine all the ingredients apart from the pine nuts until smooth.
2. Spread over your meat dish.
3. Perhaps sprinkle pine nuts over the top.
4. Bake at 180°C for 15 minutes until the top is going golden.

Sauces for meat dishes

Fruit sauces for meat dishes

1. Take any fruit, or combination of, that you like, from apple and apricots to black-currants and blackberries, plums and pears.
2. Boil up gently until they go soft.
3. Mash.
4. If too runny, add coconut flour until you get the right consistency.

Spicy sauces

Horseradish – grate and mix with thick coconut milk.
Ginger – ditto.
Garlic – ditto.
All improve with keeping in the fridge.

Herb sauces

1 Cut up your favourite herbs – this works well with mint, sage, rosemary and tarragon.
2. Pack into a small pot and fill with cider vinegar and a pinch of Sunshine salt.
3. Leave to infuse.

You are now well on your way to becoming a PK cook. As Craig's Nan used to say to him, when giving advice on possible brides:

'Kissing don't last; cookery do.'
In fact, Nan Robinson was quoting George Meredith, English novelist and poet,
12 February 1828 – 18 May 1909,
from his novel *The Ordeal of Richard Feverel* (1859)

P.S. from Craig – I ended up with a bride who could do both very well!

Chapter 13

PK salads, coleslaws and dressings

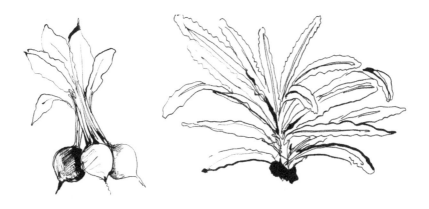

The word 'salad' derives from the Latin *sal* (salt), a form of which is *salata* (salted things). In classical times, raw vegetables were eaten with salt and always with a dressing of vinegar or oil and this dish was called 'salata'. The inclusion of an oil to the 'salads' of the Romans and Greeks gives us a first clue as to how modern salads should be prepared.

Another clue comes from Lucius Junius Moderatus Columella (4 – 70 AD), generally regarded as the most important writer on agriculture in the Roman empire, who, in his 12-volume *Res Rustica*, recommends the inclusion of eggs and nuts in 'salata'.

I routinely ask my patients about their diet. Invariably the comment 'Well, I eat lots of salad' is accompanied by a smug smile. Oh dear... I am going to have to disillusion you. Salads may satisfy your palate and conscience, but they will not satisfy your appetite. One cannot be well nourished by salad alone. Modern Western salads not only lack fuel in the form of fibre and fat, but they also lack goodness in the form of protein and micronutrients. We have salad vegetables not to nourish us, but to entertain us with that crunch factor.*

So, the redeeming features of salad are taste and texture – variety and crunch are satisfying and enhance the eating experience. I cannot tell the difference between salads and coleslaws – contents vary simply with the time of the year. They both derive from chopped raw veg, vary according to what is available and which dressing is used: French dressing, mayonnaise or hollandaise.

Table 13.1: PK salad ingredients

Green leaves	Lettuce (dozens of varieties), rocket, parsley, land cress, chicory, watercress, spinach, kale, endive, Japanese greens
Cabbage and cabbage family	Red, white, green Sprouts, kale, purple sprouting, Swiss chard Grated kohl rabi
Sauerkraut	See page 157
Green beans	Mangetout, French beans, broad beans, peas
Asparagus	
Alliums	Onions (red and white), leeks, shallots
Root veg	Grated carrot, beetroot, celeriac
Herbs	Marjoram, coriander, thyme, sage, rosemary, mint, cress

* The importance of the crunch factor in our enjoyment of eating has been confirmed in a 2015 paper by Charles Spence, called 'Eating with our ears'. Spence looked at the crispiness and crunchiness of many food types, from salads to bacons to the crackle that one senses when drinking sparkling water, and he even went on to investigate the distinctive 'cracking' sound at the first bite of the Magnum Ice Cream – when a new formula was tried for Magnum, which reduced this cracking sound, sales fell dramatically! I am not suggesting Magnum Ice Cream in your diet, but the point remains that sounds are important in the taste and eating experience and salads provide this 'crunch'.

Pickles	Onions, gherkins, olives, beetroot, jalapenos, artichokes
Summer salad	Tomato, cucumber, green/red/yellow peppers, celery, radish, spring onions
Fruit	Avocado, grated apple
PK nuts	Walnuts, Brazils, pecans, almonds – see Appendix 3 for carb content
PK seeds	Sunflower, pumpkin, sesame – see Appendix 3 for carb content
Eggs or meat	Corned beef, chunks of salami, cold meat
Biltong, pork scratchings	
Fish or shellfish	Anchovies, sardines, mackerel, salmon (tinned, fresh or frozen – I usually use tinned) Prawns, shrimps, cockles, mussels (tinned, fresh or frozen)
Smoked fish	
Quorn or tofu	
Vegan cheese	Cheddar, feta, mozzarella-like

Salad dressings

Always make a large batch because PK dressings keep so well. Put any of the options listed in Table 13.2 into a lidded jar, shake it up and store it in the fridge.

Table 13.2: Essentials for French dressing, mayonnaise and hollandaise

Essentials for French dressing	Large slug of oil	In order of preference, I use olive, hemp, rapeseed, safflower and sesame oils; all must be cold-pressed virgins... ho ho... to go with the brothels – see Chapter 3 (page 42)
	Same amount of freshly squeezed lemon or lime juice	
	Same amount of cider, white or red wine vinegar	Be sure you are not yeast allergic
	Garlic – at least 1 clove; usually 3 or 4, crushed (I love garlic)	Very Lazy Garlic is quicker but not quite so good!
	Dollop of sunflower lecithin	This emulsifies and blends the oil and water components to a thick gloop
	Large pinch Sunshine salt to provide all essential minerals, vitamin D and vitamin B12. Pepper	Shake it all up together
Extras	Teaspoon grain mustard...	...or horseradish sauce or grated fresh ginger
	If you are well within your carb allowance...	...then a ½ teaspoon of treacle imparts great texture
To make mayonnaise	Add in 2 egg yolks	Whizz it all up together
To make hollandaise	Instead of egg yolk, dollop of Grace coconut milk	Whizz it all up together

Michelle's very quick mayonnaise

Egg yolk, raw
Lemon juice and/or cider vinegar
1 dollop coconut cream
Sunshine salt[†]

Whiz up the raw egg yolk with the lemon juice/cider vinegar), coconut cream and a pinch of salt.

The Golden Rule

The Golden Rule is to keep it quick, simple and easy. I am idle and I expect the rest of you to be so too. If you are challenged by energy, time or inclination, then buy prepared salads,[‡] pour on hemp oil and generously sprinkle with Sunshine salt.

[†] The iodine in Sunshine salt gives the mayonnaise a darker colour; if I'm ever making it for the unconverted I use plain sea salt.

[‡] **Point of historical interest:** Virgil (70 - 19 BC) wrote briefly about the preparation of salads in his work *Moretum*. He says:

It manus in gyrum; paullatim singula vires
Deperdunt proprias; color est E pluribus unus.
or
'Spins round the stirring hand; lose by degrees
Their separate powers the parts, and comes at last,
From many several colours, one that rules'

So, the motto of the United States of America, *E pluribus unus*, is in fact an instruction in a salad recipe!

Chapter 14

Puddings, sweets and sweeteners

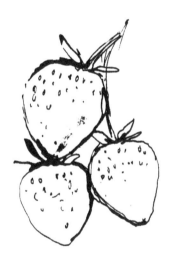

Did I catch you out? If you find yourself turning straight to this chapter, then you have failed the keto test – you are still a sugar and carb addict. I have been through the full evolution of using various sweeteners and have come to the conclusion that none are permitted.

thy sweet deceiving,
Lock me in delight awhile.

John Fletcher, 1579 – 1625, playwright

This is how it is with sweeteners; they 'deceive' us through a variety of means, which we often perceive as a 'delight', and here the addiction begins and continues. So, sweeteners, real or artificial, must be used with great circumspection for three reasons:

1. Whether real, natural (e.g. xylitol, stevia) or artificial (e.g. saccharine or aspartame), they prevent the palate from changing away from craving sweetness. But change it can, will and does. One such example is the sugar addict who has successfully, and for some time, stopped sweetening his tea – now any sugar taste in his tea seems disgustingly sweet. I find I can now eat blackcurrants (admittedly with coconut milk) without my mouth puckering up with the sharpness; for me this is a real change. A sweet taste hit switches on a sugar craving in the same way that the whiff of tobacco smoke may switch on the desire for a fag in nicotine addicts. We all know that smokers have to stop smoking completely – they cannot be satisfied with one puff a day. The same is true of alcoholics – they celebrate complete abstinence because they know this is the only way to cure their addiction. They have no 'off' button so do not dare switch it 'on'.

2. **The Pavlovian*response:** The body is intelligent. It knows that a sugar hit will require an insulin spike to deal with it. It has learned this from experience, and so anticipates the sugar spike from a sweet taste in the mouth and pours out insulin in response to such. Artificial sweeteners will therefore spike insulin and switch off fat burning and so push you back into the metabolic hinterland (where there is no fuel available from carbs and you cannot burn fat because insulin is high – see page xx). This explains why artificial sweeteners are so counter-productive in calorie restricted diets.

3. Artificial sweeteners are toxic in their own right. Aspartame is metabolised in the liver to formaldehyde, a neurotoxin and indeed a pesticide. I remain convinced that a 39-year-old lady who consulted me had her motor neurone disease triggered

---

* **Historical note:** Ivan Pavlov (26 September 1849 – 27 February 1936) played the sound of a metronome to dogs and afterwards gave them food. After a few repetitions, the dogs associated the noise of the metronome with food and so would salivate merely on the sound of the metronome even in the absence of food. This is much like rustling a packet of crisps at Craig – he will salivate! Pavlov went on to report more observations about this 'Pavlovian response'; for example, the 'conditioning' happened more quickly when the interval between the sound of the metronome and the food was shortest during the initial period when the dogs were being 'conditioned'.

by a diet which saw her replace all sweeteners with aspartame; we reckoned she had consumed over a kilogram of aspartame during a few months. This is the youngest case of MND I have ever seen. Aspartame is also a carcinogen. To quote Rycerz and Jaworska-Adamu (2013): 'Despite intense speculations about the carcinogenicity of aspartame, the latest studies show that its metabolite, diketo-piperazine, is carcinogenic in the CNS. It contributes to the formation of tumours in the CNS such as gliomas, medulloblastomas and meningiomas.'[1]

When people tell me they do not like a particular food, I ask them to analyse what they mean by 'like'. The answer should relate to taste, texture (crunch or chew factors) or smell (something familiar or evocative). However, many people 'like' a food because it provides a psychological hit. They are often unaware of this mechanism and refuse psychologically to admit to such. Without a sugar or carb rush, the meal does not satisfy. Take the sugar rush out and junk food reverts to the bland, tasteless, nutritionally criminal mush that it is.

PK puddings[†] and treats

While puddings are generally not compatible with being in ketosis, if you keep your eye on your carb consumption (see Appendix 3), and your ketone levels with your breathom-eter, the following may work as part of your diet. In addition to the recipe ideas below, see Chapter 9: The PK dairy, for cream, ice cream and PK chocolates and remember my favourite standby – berries, fresh or frozen, with coconut cream.

[†] **Literary aside:** The English language is a wonderful thing. 'Pudding' is what some would call the 'dessert' course of the meal. Others might call it the 'sweet' course or 'afters'. Puddings can also be savoury as in 'black pudding' or 'Yorkshire pudding' but, unless qualified by a term denoting a savoury meal, pudding is taken as referring to a 'sweet' dish in the UK and Commonwealth countries.

Michelle's chia seed and sunflower cream

This makes an unusual but beautiful, dairy-free ice cream

Chia seeds
Sunflower seeds
Water

1. Soak the chia seeds the night or morning before until all burst open and become super-gelatinous, resembling frogs' spawn slightly.
2. Soak the sunflower seeds in enough water to cover them for 6-12 hours/overnight. Then strain off the water, washing them through a sieve.
3. Pop the sunflower seeds with the chia seeds into the Nutribullet.
4. Top up with water so that it looks like it is double water to seeds in the bullet. The amount of water depends how runny you want your cream; if you want it thick, add less water. However, too little water and it will be too thick to blend, too much and it will be very runny and too watery, but you can always add more if too runny. Trial and error works best for this one!
5. Once blended, scoop into a bowl or jug depending on the consistency and serve up with a bowl of summer berries, or stewed rhubarb – a wonderful combination.

Crumble topping

This is a great topping for stewed fruit (berries, apples, cooking pears). Use equal amounts of the ingredients listed:

Coconut flour
Almond flour
Desiccated coconut
Sesame seeds
Coconut oil

1. Preheat your oven to 160°C (not too hot or it burns).
2. Put equal amounts of coconut flour, almond flour, desiccated coconut, sesame

seeds and coconut oil in a bowl.
3. Use your hands to mix it all together to a crumbly texture.
4. Sprinkle it evenly over your choice of stewed fruit.
5. Bake in the oven for 20-30 minutes until it browns.

Easy chocolate mousse

225 g/8 oz good-quality plain 85% chocolate
25 g/1 oz coconut oil (or butter)
1-2 tsp instant coffee granules (optional)
4 eggs, separated
Few drops vanilla essence

1. Place the chocolate, oil/butter and coffee, if using, in a heatproof bowl and place over a saucepan of hot water. Leave to melt, stirring occasionally, until smooth.
2. Remove the bowl from over the pan of hot water and stir in the egg yolks and vanilla essence. (For a richer taste, add in couple of tablespoons of brandy or coffee or orange liqueur.)
3. In a clean, dry bowl, whisk the egg whites until stiff.
4. Using a large metal spoon, gently fold a quarter of the egg whites into the chocolate mixture then continue a quarter at a time until all the egg white is mixed in.
5. When just evenly combined, spoon into cold serving dishes and place in the refrigerator for 30-60 minutes.

Coconut brownies

100 g coconut oil
100 g 90% dark chocolate
2 eggs
1 tsp vanilla essence
Pinch Sunshine salt
30 g coconut flour
200 g vegan cream cheese, chopped into bite-sized pieces

1. Preheat the oven to 180°C/350°F.
2. Grease an oven-proof dish.
3. Melt the oil and chocolate together over a low heat; when melted, set aside to cool.
4. In a large bowl, whisk together the eggs, vanilla and salt.
5. When smooth, whisk in the chocolate until well combined.
6. Gently stir through the coconut flour, one tablespoon at a time.
7. Place half of the brownie batter into the prepared oven-proof dish.
8. Top with the chopped cream cheese and finally spread over the other half of the brownie batter. You want your mixture to be about an inch thick.
9. Place into the oven for 20 minutes or until cooked to your liking.
10. Remove from the oven, cool and serve.

Michelle's cordyceps and carob-flour chocolates

These make a lovely little treat to have after dinner.

¼ cup cocoa butter
¼ cup coconut oil
I dsp cordyceps powder
I dsp carob flour, or cocoa powder if more of a kick is wanted
Nuts for sprinkling – pecans, macadamia, Brazils are lowest in carbs
Desiccated coconut for sprinkling

1. Melt the cocoa butter with the coconut oil over a low heat.
2. Add the cordyceps powder and carob flour or cocoa powder.
3. Add the nuts of choice, and desiccated coconut if using. (Try to avoid high-carb cashews and pistachios.)
4. Pour into a square container layered in baking paper and pop into the fridge until cooled.
5. Take out and cut into small squares.

Carolyn's special chocolate

This is how to turn boring dark chocolate into something more artisanal...

200 g 85-90% dark chocolate
10-15 drops peppermint essential oil

1. Melt the chocolate very gently over a pan of hot water.
2. Take off the heat and stir in the peppermint oil.
3. Pour onto a sheet of 'If You Care' or similar baking parchment on top of a large baking tray.
4. Sprinkle some de-hulled hemp seeds over.
5. Pop in the freezer for an hour to set.
6. Break into pieces and then keep in the fridge (as thinner than a bar of chocolate, it may slightly melt at room temperature).

My favourite (but pricier) substitutes for the peppermint oil and seeds are:
- 1 drop rose essential oil, and when poured onto the baking parchment, top with toasted flaked almonds
- Orange essential oil (5 drops) and spices
- Lemon essential oil and cardamom.

Chapter 15

PK snacks

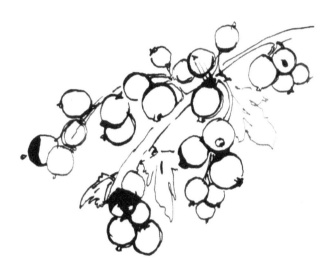

In recent times, 'snacks' have become an almost 'expected' part of the Western daily diet as this reflects the carbohydrate addiction. Internet memes abound vis: 'Keep your friends close, and your snacks closer.' For the addict, snacks it seems are more important than friends.

Remember that once keto-adapted, although you may feel a bit peckish and deserving of a snack, you will not feel that awful energy dip that the carb addict will if s/he misses her/his snack. Please do take care with snacks and do stick to the calorie and protein intakes described in Chapter 3. Snacks should be a treat, and not used as a *necessity* between meals.

No-preparation snacks

Low-carb nuts and seeds such as Brazils, pecans, coconut flakes
Salami, pork scratchings, biltong
Olives

Michelle's linseed biscuits

I cup golden linseeds
Water, a little
I egg
Coconut oil or lard, a dollop
Seeds, whole, such as sunflower, pumpkin, sesame
Desiccated coconut (optional)
Carob powder (optional)

1. Grind the linseeds in your Nutribullet or equivalent.
2. Mix with a tad of the water, add the egg and the coconut oil or lard.
3. Mix in your choice of other seeds, coconut, and perhaps carob powder.
4. Dollop the mixture in between 'sandwich' sheets of baking paper and use a rolling pin to flatten to the thickness of a finger.
5. Peel off the top layer of baking paper.
6. Cook in the oven at about 150°C for half an hour until crispy on the top and slightly soft in the middle.
7. Serve hot with butter or coconut oil.

Sue McCullagh's seed balls – mother's mainstay!

I dollop coconut oil
I dollop ghee
Sunshine salt
Seeds
Nuts

1. Melt the coconut oil and ghee together in a saucepan and add a healthy sprinkling of Sunshine salt.
2. Grind a similar amount of the seeds and nuts in your Nutribullet/equivalent and add to the melted fats.
3. Let the mixture go semi-cold so that you can form it into balls; put these into mini cake casings and pop them into the freezer OR just pour the mixture into a square container lined with baking paper and cool in the fridge. Once cold and fully set, cut into small squares and freeze.
4. Both the balls and squares can be eaten straight from freezer as a delicious snack.

Garlic and rosemary linseed crisp breads

These can be made in large batches and frozen. They are delicious as a starter with liver or fish paté, or as a lunch-time snack.

I cup linseed
I tbsp chia seeds
I clove garlic, mashed
Handful rosemary leaves
I tsp Sunshine salt
Water, a little

1. Grind the linseed and chia seeds in your Nutribullet/equivalent.
2. Add the garlic and rosemary leaves and grind up in your Nutribullet/blender with a good teaspoon of Sunshine salt.
3. Transfer to a bowl and add a little water until it is soft enough to make a dough.

4. Put the dough between two sheets of greaseproof paper and roll out to about 1-2 mm thick, so super-thin.
5. Peel off the top sheet and pop in the oven on a low heat – anything between 50 and 100°C – and let them dry out and crisp up.
6. Take out of the oven once dry and crispy and break up into biscuit-sized pieces.

Kefir cake

I cup linseeds
¼ cup coconut flour
¾ cup homemade kefir
Handful dried sour cherries, cranberries or raisins
I dsp ghee
I dsp pig or beef fat

1. Grind the linseed in your Nutribullet/equivalent until it is a powder.
2. Add the coconut flour.
3. Pour in the kefir until you achieve a dough-like consistency.
4. Add the dried fruit; this will expand so the mixture becomes slightly lighter and fluffier.
5. Leave in the fridge for two days for the sugars to ferment in the fruit.
6. Pre-heat the oven to 200°C.
7. Remove the dough from the fridge and fold in the ghee and pig or beef fat
8. Line a dish with baking paper, dollop the mixture in the centre and press it in to fill the dish.
9. Cook in the oven for 40 minutes, or until brown and crispy on top.

Wendy Cresswell's hard tack

Wendy never fails to join us on our annual long-distance cross-Wales ride. Her recipe below is well tested and never fails to satisfy.

4 handfuls nuts, blitzed
I cup linseed made into flour
Handful currants, blitzed
½ cup coconut oil, melted

1. Blitz all the ingredients together in a food processor.
2. Press the mixure into a Tupperware-type container.
3. Put this in the fridge to set hard.
4. Then cut into squares; once cut it doesn't melt easily.
5. Variations: You can add to/change the ingredients around but keep the linseed and oil constant.

Miso kale crisps

150 g kale or cavolo nero
I tbsp pale (shiro) miso (or wasabi ½ tbsp)
2 tbsp rice vinegar
2 tbsp melted coconut oil
I tbsp togarashi or furikake spice mix

1. Preheat the oven to 150°C/130°C fan /Gas 2.
2. Prepare the kale or cavolo nero – use big leaves of kale; remove the stems and then rip or cut the leaves into coarse pieces of approximately 5 x 5 cm. (The pre-cut bags include the tough woody stems, so avoid those as the stems don't crisp like the leaves.)
3. In a large bowl, mix the miso, rice vinegar and coconut oil together.
4. Add the kale/cavolo nero leaves to the miso mixture and massage it into the leaves.
5. Place the kale in a single layer on a large baking tray or two smaller ones.
6. Sprinkle the spice mix over it and bake for 20 minutes or until crisp.

Angie Jones's fruit leathers

These quantities make two sheets of 24 x 30 cm

500 g total of plums, blackberries and/or blackcurrants, raspberries, blueberries (whatever is in the garden)
500 g peeled, cored and chopped cooking apples (2-3 large apples)
Juice of 1 lemon
Up to 150 g honey (the less the better – I do not use any at all)

1. Preheat the oven to a very low setting – 60°C/Gas mark 1/8 approx *or* use a dehydrator.
2. Put the berries, apple and lemon juice into a pan.
3. Cook gently until soft and pulpy, which should take about 20 minutes.
4. Rub the mixture through a sieve or mouli into a bowl; you should have about 700 g smooth fruit purée.
5. Add the honey (if you must!) and mix well.
6. Line two baking sheets, measuring about 24 x 30 cm, with baking parchment.
7. Divide the puree between the two baking sheets; spread it out lightly with the back of a spoon until the puree covers the sheets in a thin, even layer.
8. Put the baking sheets in the oven (or dehydrator) and leave for 12-18 hours, until the fruit puree is completely dry and peels off the parchment easily.
9. Roll up the leathers in greaseproof paper and store in an airtight tin.
10. Use within a few months – mine never last that long!

Variations:

Spicing the purée with a little cinnamon.

Use peaches.

Infuse the leathers with a few honeysuckle blossoms as they cook.

For savoury leathers try using half apple and half tomato seasoned with 2 tsp of celery salt.

Pork scratchings

If any food should be a 'super food' this is it. When you purchase large chunks of leaf fat, you are not just buying lard. You are also buying peritoneal membranes which hold it all together alongside lymph nodes and lymphatics. These latter items are highly nutritious and make for the most divine scratchings.

1. Cut the leaf fat into date-sized pieces and put into a saucepan.
2. Cook on a low heat so they just bubble a little and until the scratchings are brown and the fat still white. Watchout! It is very easy to over-cook them at the last moment.
3. Pour the white fat into your dripping pot.
4. Sprinkle Sunshine salt on the scratchings and watch those happy children devour them!

Note from Sarah: In my family, major wars would erupt if the distribution of scratchings was not seen to be entirely fair. We would all oversee the division of them into four equal piles. We would then pick straws for who took which pile. The next stage of proceedings was to savour each mouthful and see who could eat them the slowest, and then tease the eater-uppers with that final delicious mouthful. One ploy would be to secret a morsel without the others noticing… then triumphantly reveal this when all else had been consumed. Indeed, we used this same method to split up the contents of our mum's house, after she died, into four heaps. It resulted in a hilarious afternoon instead of what could have been a sombre and miserable job – I am sure she would have approved.

Note from Craig: In our house things are much more sedate, due to there being two resident mathematicians. For dividing into two equal piles, for example, the procedure is that one person divides the food into two piles and the other person chooses which pile they want. This encourages the 'divider' to divide equally. More complicated methods, from set theory, apply for dividing into three and four piles. Amazingly, I and daughter, Gina, normally end up with bigger piles than Penny and our son, Conor, but it is all done completely fairly according to set theory… those who are interested may like to read https://en.wikipedia.org/wiki/Fair_cake-cutting although cakes are most definitely not 'PK'!

Chapter 16

Herbs and spices

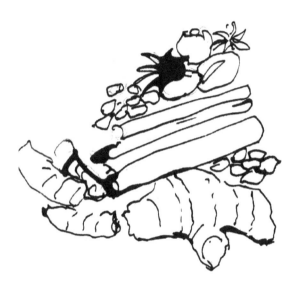

Life is an arms race. You and I represent a potential free lunch for the myriad of bacteria, moulds, parasites, worms, yeasts and viruses which are constantly straining to make themselves at home in our secure, warm, moist, comfortable bodies. Throughout Evolution, infections have been major killers. We imagine we have won that arms race with modern hygiene, antimicrobials, drugs and vaccinations. Wrong! We have been lulled into a false sense of security by drug company propaganda. We know that low-grade chronic infections are driving many chronic pathologies, such as autoimmunity (one in 20 Westerners have an autoimmune condition), allergy, arthritis, heart disease, dementia and cancer. See our book *The Infection Game* for more detail.

The principles of prevention and treatment are to starve out the microbes with a ketogenic diet and then kill them all which ways. Herbs and spices are very useful weapons. If you look at life from the point of view of a plant, it does not want to be eaten. Plants cannot run away like prey animals; their only defence is to make themselves as unpalatable as possible. All plants are stuffed with natural antimicrobials: antihelminthics, antiparasitics, antibacterials, antifungals and antivirals. Indeed, if any plant were lacking any such antimicrobials, it would have been overcome by infection at some point in Evolution. Plants too are survivors of this arms race. Many gorgeous Indian spices have been adopted by humans to preserve food between harvesting and eating when it may otherwise go off in a hot climate. Consuming such further assists us humans to keep microbial invaders at bay.

> *Bernard was right; the pathogen is nothing; the terrain is everything.*
> The last words of Louis Pasteur, 1822 – 1895*

What is so fascinating is that the body knows what it needs for health. The science is call pharmacognosy – the study of plants and other natural sources for medicines; the mechanism has yet to be worked out, but the practical reality is that we are attracted to those remedies by 'likes'. Once addiction has been overcome, smell and taste draw us to the correct healing herbs, spices, foods and perhaps clays. If you like it, it is doing good. So, the key to good health and cooking is to use those ingredients which smell and taste great to you. Furthermore, these preferences are peculiar to individuals and conditions – they are personal. I loved Caroline Ingraham's book *Animal Self-medication* which describes 'zoo-pharmacognosy' – how the rest of the animal kingdom chooses its own remedies.[1] Interested readers are also referred to *Really Wild Remedies—Medicinal Plant Use by Animals* by Jennifer A. Biser of the Smithsonian National Zoological Park, USA. Biser describes how local people learn remedies from animals:

---

* **Historical note:** The French scientist Louis Pasteur was the originator of the 'germ theory' that disease has a microbial origin. His rival, Claude Bernard (1813 – 1878), believed that the 'terrain' (the underlying health of the human body) was more important than the infective organism (the pathogen) and medicine should concentrate on strengthening the body to fight off disease.

In Tanzania's Mahale Mountains National Park, a lethargic chimpanzee suffering from diarrhea and malaise slowly pulls a young shoot off a small tree called Vernonia amygdalina. *She peels away the shoot's bark and leaves with her teeth, and begins chewing on the succulent pith. Swallowing the juice, she spits out most of the fibers, then continues to chew and swallow a few more stalks for half an hour.*

Nearby, pausing only to wipe the feverish sweat from her brow, the WaTongwe woman finishes crushing a few leaves and stems a fellow tribe member brought her from the mujonso, or "bitter leaf", tree. She soaks them in a bowl of cold water while her stomach aches with a dull pain. Closing her eyes and grimacing in anticipation of the liquid's foul taste, she holds her nose and gulps down the bitter elixir, hoping this reliable remedy will rid her of the intestinal pain that's plagued her for days. Recovered within 24 hours, both of these females resume business as usual. They were both suffering the effects of an intestinal parasite infection. And, in case you haven't guessed, they both ate from the same tree.[2]

Which herbs and spices to use

I do not think it matters much which you use so long as you use those that you like, and lots of them. Everyone will have their own personal list, but my favourites are shown in Table 16.1.

Table 16.1: Recommended herbs and when to use them

Food	What to add	Comments
Meat	Pepper – a lot	Pepper is a rich source of zinc and zinc deficiency is extremely common. During the 16th century pepper was a currency preferred more than gold. Indeed, even earlier than that pepper was highly valued: Alaric I (King of the Visigoths) and Attila (Ruler of the Huns) both demanded a ransom of black pepper in order to stop attacking Rome in the 5th century. There is even a mortgage lender in the UK called 'Pepper Money'
	Sunshine salt	This supplies all essential minerals for the immune system to fight invaders. See chapter 17

Food	What to add	Comments
	Garlic – a lot	Garlic supplements are the most consumed supplement in Germany due to its multiple health benefits; it is especially protective against heart and arterial disease
• Lamb	Cook with a large handful of rosemary	Rosemary is antibacterial and antioxidant. A long-living community on the Greek island of Ikaria, who have no Alzheimer's, attribute their longevity to living on a hillside (exercise) and rosemary[3]
• Pork	Berries, plums, apple	The sharpness of these sauces is an exquisite contrast and balance to the fat of pork (see Chapter 12: Main courses)
• Beef	Horseradish[†] sauce and wasabi	Both have good anti-cancer properties
PK butter	Garlic	To make garlic bread… yum, yum!
Curry dishes	Ginger	A medicinal spice widely used in Chinese medicine
	Cardamon, cumin, coriander, cinnamon… many more	Buy the best you can get, keep them whole and grind at the last minute. Roll the raw lump of meat in the spices and flash fry them – this releases the best flavours
Salads	Rocket, land cress, coriander, marjoram, tarragon, sage, mint, basil	Combine these with whatever is in the garden at that time of year
PK bread	1 tsp caraway, cumin, fennel seed	
All vegetable dishes	Pour on lots of cold-pressed olive oil	or any other cold-pressed nut, seed or vegetable oil you like
Onions and leeks	Turmeric powder sprinkled on – a lot	Curcumin is the active ingredient of turmeric and widely used in many gut conditions as an anti-inflammatory

[†] Why 'horseradish'? In German, it is called meerrettich (sea radish) because it grows by the sea. Possibly, the English mispronounced the German word meer and began calling it '"mareradish'. Eventually it became known as horseradish, with the understanding of 'mare' as an adult female horse. Yes, English is a wonderful language!

Cabbage	Caraway seeds	
Crumble toppings	Cinnamon - a lot Nutmeg, allspice	All are anti-inflammatory, improve brain function and are anti-cancer
Tea...	Black tea, green tea Ginger tea	Herbal teas have antimicrobial properties and help keep the upper gut 'clean and tidy'
...and coffee	...but do not over-do these – limit tea (3 normal-sized cups) or coffee (3 small cups) and don't drink either after midday as this can upset sleep	Improves brain function in the short term

Good antimicrobials and great taste

- Rhodiola tea – is reputed to have activity against retroviruses. Pour boiling water over 1 tsp.
- Astragalus dried root – this can be eaten off the spoon and chewed until all the flavour has gone, then spit out the woody remains. It makes a reasonable chewing gum substitute. It is also delicious in stews – you can add in tablespoon amounts.
- Cordyceps makes the most delicious chocolate. It imparts a flavour which tastes like chocolate with a hint of coffee and truffle. It really is quite superb – one of the best medicines ever! Here is the recipe.

Cordyceps chocolate

200 g cocoa butter fat
200 g coconut oil
200 g cordyceps powder
200 g dried goji berries

1. Put the cocoa butter fat, coconut oil and cordyceps powder into a pan to melt the oils and mix in the cordceps powder.
2. Tip the goji berries into a flat plastic container. (As an alternative my daughter uses lots of paper cake cups.)

3. Cover the berries with the mix and put in the fridge to set.
4. Eat directly from cold.

Persian seven-spice garam masala recipe from Dr Shideh Puria

One can make various modifications to this recipe according to one's taste but this is how I do it. It is an incredibly useful mix which can be used for vegetable dishes or rice dishes (including cauliflower rice) or to flavour meat, especially lamb chops.

150 g coriander seeds
180 g black peppercorns (for a milder flavour white peppercorns could work too)
150 g cinnamon (not cassia) sticks
130 g cumin seeds
120 g allspice berries
40 g cloves
40 g whole nutmeg
And for the extra Persian touch, 20 g Persian dried rose buds
Other options:
30 g cardamom seeds
20 g dried ginger
20 g fennel seeds

1. Mill all the ingredients in a powerful blender like a Vitamix to make a fragrant flour.
2. Keep in a glass jar with a lid; the mix will keep for a year plus.

Chapter 17

PK salt

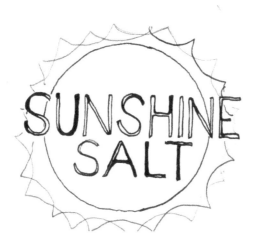

---

* Historical footnote: This is the earliest publication of the phrase 'salt of the earth' in the English language (circa 1386). Geoffrey Chaucer (c.1343 – 25 October 1400) is often known as the Father of English literature, and was the first poet to be buried in 'Poets' Corner' at Westminster Abbey. Salary derives from the Latin *salarium* which has the root 'sal', or 'salt'. There is much debate about the reasons as to why 'sal' is the root. The most oft-quoted link is referenced from Pliny the Elder, who stated, as an aside in his *Natural History*, that 'In

Essential salts

Athletes are very aware of the importance of electrolytes ('salts' or 'minerals' – same thing!). They are lost with intensive exercise through sweating and in urine. Athletes are careful to replace sodium salt, but they forget the micro-minerals. The point here is that sweat is simply blood minus the solid bits (red cells, white cells, platelets and various proteins). All minerals are lost, and therefore a true electrolyte mix should include all minerals. Indeed, there are increasing reports of top athletes dropping dead with exercise. I suspect one unrecognised cause is acute magnesium (Mg)[†] deficiency. The link between sudden death and magnesium deficiency has long been known, as is evident from the 1992 paper by MJ Eisenberg in the *American Heart Journals*: As he stated, much evidence in the 30 years prior to this publication, from epidemiological studies and autopsies to clinical and animal studies, suggested a strong link between magnesium deficiency and sudden death. Links found included sudden death being more common in areas with water supplies of low magnesium content, myocardial magnesium content being low in people who had suffered sudden death, and cardiac arrhythmias and coronary artery vasospasms being caused by a deficiency in magnesium. Indeed, it 'works the other way' as well - namely, that giving intravenous magnesium reduces the risk of arrhythmia and death after acute myocardial infarction (heart attack).

With running, one loses about 10 mg of magnesium per mile through sweat and urine. Calcium is necessary for heart muscle to contract; magnesium for it to relax. Exercise can induce an acute magnesium deficiency so that the heart stops in systole (when the

---

Rome... the soldier's pay was originally salt and the word salary derives from it...'.[1] Other newer sources state that Roman soldiers were paid in coins, and that the word 'salarium' is derived from the word 'sal' because a soldier may have been required by Army regulations to buy salt for his diet with some of said coins. Yet more sources state that the use of 'sal' as a root of 'salarium' derives from the price in coins that had to be paid by the Roman Empire to have soldiers conquer salt supplies and guard the Salt Roads ('Via Salaria') that led to Rome. Even more intriguingly, some historians think that the word 'soldier' itself derives from the Latin 'sal dare' (to give salt), although I was taught that the word 'soldier' derives from the Latin for gold, 'solidus', with which soldiers were known to have been paid. Craig, via Mr Ferris, my Latin Master.

[†] **Historical note:** Magnesium is a paramagnetic metal – i.e. it is slightly attracted by a magnet. The Latin root is from 'Magnes', the Shepherd Boy, who was reported by Pliny the Elder to have been the accidental discoverer of magnetism. Pliny writes: 'Nicander is our authority that it [magnetite ore] was called Magnes, from the man who first discovered it on Mount Ida, and he is said to have found it when the nails of his shoes and the ferrule of his staff adhered to it, as he was pasturing his herds.' So said Nicander of Colophon, a Greek poet, physician and grammarian. (Thanks again are due to Mr Ferris – it is a wonder we did any 'real' study! Craig.)

ventricles are contracting) – it does not have sufficient magnesium to relax. Postmortem findings are normal, because this is a functional problem not an anatomical one.

Western diets are mineral-deficient for several reasons:

1. We no longer recycle human sewerage onto the fields. There is a net movement of minerals from the soil, into plants, then animals, then us …but we throw them away. This means the mineral content of soils and foods has declined progressively since the 1950s. This is not my opinion but shown by Government figures. Figure 17.1 shows the data for the US.[1] In the UK, a paper by AM Mayer in the *British Food Journal* in 1992 recorded that, in the 20 vegetables studied, there were statistically significant reductions in the levels of calcium, magnesium, copper and sodium of up to 25% between 1930 and 1980 and it can only have worsened since then.[2] Even organic food is micronutrient-deficient compared with the ideal because of the failure to recycle which also applies.

Parts per million

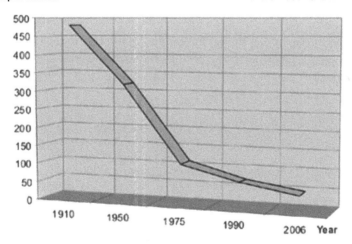

Figure 17.1: A graph showing soil mineral depletion in the United States since 1910 (source: US Dept of Agriculture.[1])

2. Modern Western diets based on sugars and refined carbohydrates may be rich in calories but are markedly deficient in micronutrients. Many micronutrients are stripped out in the refining process. I have yet to see normal tests of micronutrient

status in someone eating a Western diet who is not taking supplements.

3. We are no longer physically active and do not need to eat large amounts of food. Less food means fewer micronutrients.
4. Our requirements for micronutrients are increasing because we live in an increasingly toxic world and we need micronutrients to detoxify. This is magnified by the upper fermenting gut which does not absorb nutrients as it should (see Chapter 1).
5. Sunshine is considered to be a danger to health. Our sun phobia has resulted in widespread vitamin D deficiency and this is contributing to epidemics of osteoporosis, cancer and heart disease.

There is much more detail in our book *Ecological Medicine*.

The PK diet goes some way to addressing the above issues, but Sunshine salt is an essential addition. It should be used in cooking and on food to secure our intake of essential minerals. A further joy of Sunshine salt is that a reluctant family can be effectively treated without resorting to coercion and bullying. I was once caught out by my daughters when I experimented with B vitamins in bread – the loaf turned out bright yellow.

The bottom line is we should all be consuming 5 grams (a rounded teaspoonful) of Sunshine salt daily. In addition to vitamin D, this contains all essential minerals permitted as food additives, in a form that can be absorbed and in the correct proportion. This will supply you with the following:

Table 17.1: Essential minerals and their availability in Sunshine salt

Essential mineral	Amount in 5 g Sunshine salt	For the man on the Clapham omnibus*	For the boffin – this mineral is essential:
Maldon sea salt (sodium chloride or NaCl)	4 g	Salt is much maligned nowadays, but it is an essential part of our diet; it was recognised by the Ancients as essential.‡ The need for salt increases when in ketosis	For: • hydration • energy delivery • kidney function. Sea salt contains other essential trace minerals in miniscule amounts, insufficient for normal human needs, so it must be reinforced with other minerals

Calcium chloride (CaCl)	60 mg	This amount of calcium is lower than the RDA (recommended daily allowance) but the extra vitamin D in Sunshine salt greatly enhances its absorption	For: • muscle contraction (including heart muscle) • nerve conduction • tough muscles, tendons and bones • energy delivery in the body
Magnesium chloride (MgCl)	60 mg	This amount of magnesium is lower than the RDA but the extra vitamin D in Sunshine salt greatly enhances its absorption. It is 'Nature's tranquilliser'. Mg deficiency is pandemic in Western societies. It is essential for normal heart function; deficiency is a likely cause of heart dysrhythmias and sudden death	For: • switching off muscle contraction (so allowing the heart muscle to relax) • switching off nerve excitation generated by calcium. • energy delivery in the body (mitochondria) • as a co-factor for at least 300 different enzyme systems
Potassium chloride (KCl)	40 mg	Potassium cannot be stored in the body, so you need to consume this mineral daily	For energy delivery mechanisms
Zinc chloride (ZnCl)	30 mg	Zinc deficiency is pandemic in Western societies. It helps control of blood sugar levels. Protective against heart disease and cancer. Vital for normal immunity. Deficiency in mother and therefore child is associated with dyslexia	For: • anti-infection • detox in the liver • DNA synthesis and repair • superoxide dismutase antioxidant • protein synthesis • hormone recognition

⁺ **Proverbial aside:** 'To take with a pinch of salt' in English is used to mean to take less seriously than one might otherwise. 'Pinch' is often replaced by 'grain' in American usage. First the easy bit – in old English units of weight, a grain weighed approximately 60 mg, which is about how much table salt a person might pick up between the fingers as a pinch, so a pinch and a grain weigh about the same. Next the origin: in Pliny the Elder's *Naturalis Historia* there is discussion of the discovery of a recipe for an antidote to a poison. In the antidote, one of the ingredients was a grain of salt. Consequently, this phrase soon came to mean that threats involving the poison were thus to be taken 'with a grain of salt', and therefore less seriously.

***Legal note:** The 'man on the Clapham omnibus' is a hypothetical ordinary and reasonable person, used by the courts in English law to decide whether a party has acted as a reasonable person would. If the 'man on the Clapham omnibus' would do a certain thing, or think it, then this would mean it is a reasonable action or thought. It was first put to use in the courts in a judgement by Sir Richard Henn Collins MR in 1903. He attributed it to Lord Bowen.

Essential mineral	Amount in 5 g Sunshine salt	For the man on the Clapham omnibus	For the boffin – this mineral is essential:
Iron (ferric ammonium chloride)	15 mg	Lack of iron causes anaemia	For haemoglobin which allows red cells to carry oxygen
Boron (tetraborate)	2 mg	Highly protective against arthritis	For normal calcium and magnesium metabolism
Iodine (as potassium iodate (KIO3))	1 mg	Deficiency of iodine is extremely common (estimated at over 90% of Westerners). It is needed for the synthesis of thyroid hormones; thyroid disease is estimated to affect at least 20% of Westerners. Deficiency may manifest pain, lumps and cysts	For: • synthesis of thyroid hormones • synthesis of oxytocin (the love and empathy hormone; this may be a particular problem in autism) • normal breast tissue
Manganese (Mn)	1 mg	Manganese protects against damage to energy delivery mechanisms	For the synthesis of manganese superoxide dismutase, the most important antioxidant within mitochondria
Copper (Cu)	1 mg	Copper provides links between fibres to make for tough connective tissue, muscle and bones. Deficiency can cause anaemia	For zinc/copper superoxide dismutase, a vital antioxidant outside and inside all cells
Molybdenum (Mb)	200 mcg	Molybdenum helps detox in the liver; since we live in a toxic world this function is becoming increasingly important	For the detox enzyme sulphite oxidase
Selenium (Se)	200 mcg	Selenium is highly protective against cancer and heart disease. It gives connective tissue and bone their toughness and elasticity	For glutathione peroxidase – a vital antioxidant
Chromium (C)	200 mcg	Chromium deficiency results in diabetes. It is protective against heart disease	For insulin

Vitamin D3	5000 iu	D3 deficiency is pandemic in Western sun-phobic society. D3 is highly protective against heart disease, cancer and autoimmunity. No toxicity has ever been seen in doses up to 10,000 iu daily. Being heat-stable it survives cooking	For: • enhancing the absorption of calcium and magnesium and ensuring their deposition in bone. • normal immune function – D3 is an excellent anti-inflammatory and protective against many viral infections including Covid-19
Vitamin B12	5000 mcg	B12 deficiency is pandemic in Westerners eating high-carbohydrate diets. B12 is poorly absorbed so high doses are essential; as we age and our bodies slow down our requirements for B12 increase. B12 is highly protective against heart disease, cancer and dementia. No toxicity. Being heat-stable it survives cooking	For: • healing and repair • detoxification • protein synthesis via the methylation cycle

The balance of minerals listed in Table 17.1 that make up Sunshine salt would be an excellent basis for a rehydrating mix for athletes or, indeed, people suffering from gastroenteritis. I would recommend using a rounded teaspoon in 1 litre of water (i.e. 5 grams of Sunshine salt per 1 litre of water to make a 0.05 % solution). At this dilution one can hardly taste the salt but it will be doing a power of good. (You can purchase Sunshine salt on my website: www.sales@drmyhill.co.uk.)

Chapter 18

Fermented foods

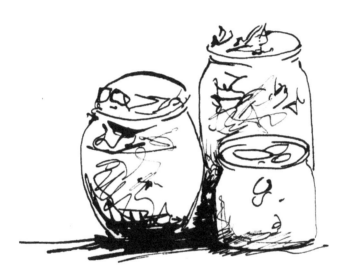

In South Korea, kimchi is eaten at breakfast, lunch and dinner, with the average South Korean eating about 150-200 grams per day in winter, and 50-100 grams in summer. Eating alone is something of a taboo in South Korea and so this tradition of eating kimchi is passed down from generation to generation, with women being slightly larger consumers. The Japanese too have fermented foods as an essential part of their daily diet. Two condiments, for example, are miso (fermented soybean paste) and soy sauce. Also, natto, made of fermented soybeans, is eaten as a standard breakfast food. Japan has the highest life expectancy in the world – 83.7 years[1] – and South Korean women have the third highest life expectancy among women at 85.5 years.[2]

The microbiome is remarkably stable and has been for generations. It is passed down through the female line much like DNA. We should inherit Mother's microbiome at the point of birth, feed it with a PK diet, then hand it on to the next generation. High-carb diets, antibiotics, micronutrient deficiencies and pollution have put paid to much of that. Consuming fermented foods may help to redress the balance.

Fermented foods may not, as we imagine, recolonise the gut with friendly microbes but they do much good in passing through:

- When foods are fermented, the sugars and starches are fermented out – so, fermented foods are necessarily low in, or devoid of, carbohydrates. You can eat fermented foods ad lib on the PK diet.
- When foods are fermented, lactic acid is produced – some sauerkrauts have a pH as low as 3.0 (the lower, the more acidic). This maintains the acidity of the stomach, so protecting against infection and improving digestion of protein and absorption of minerals. Sauerkraut is a great start to a meal because subsequent foods drop into the acid bath which kills microbes that may be present (and there will be lots in the Upper Weston kitchen).
- Lactic acid is a good food source.
- Sauerkraut is rich in vitamin K2, which is essential for normal clotting of blood and to protect against osteoporosis. We are all deficient in vitamin K – so much so that all babies are treated with vitamin K at birth to prevent haemorrhagic disease of the newborn. (See our book *Green Mother* for more details.)
- Fermented foods are high in fibre so shorten the gut transit time; consequently, potentially toxic foods spend less time in the gut (see Chapter 3).
- Fermentation is a great way of storing foods safely. If a food is teeming with friendly microbes, then the 'unfriendlies' cannot get in; this is protective against food poisoning. We know probiotics are protective against gastroenteritis.
- Fermented foods are good for educating the immune system. Microbes in them should be rapidly killed, or at least rendered inert, by stomach acid. However, these dead or inert microbes may have an important role in training and programming the immune system in the gut (and 90% of the immune system is gut-associated). The immune system is our standing army; what better way to train an army than by offering up some opposition that cannot fight back? See our book *The Infection Game*.

156

Sauerkraut

Sauerkraut is amazingly easy to make; indeed, so easy that not only can I make it but so have many other peoples. Some attention to detail is important – particularly concerning oxygen and temperature. The same technique is used to make:

Kimchi (cabbage, radish, scallion, cucumber)
Atchara in the Philippines (from papaya)
Curtido in Central America (cabbage, carrot, onion, oregano)
Dill pickles (cucumber)
Kiseli kupus in Serbia (cabbage)
Kiselo zeli in Bulgaria (cabbage)

Table 18.1: How to make sauerkraut

What to do	Notes
Weigh the vegetables	This is to get the proportion of salt correct – too much kills the friendly fermenters
Do not wash the vegetables…	…or you lose the friendly bacteria that are naturally present and essential for the fermentation
Cabbage, red or white, is the main ingredient. Cut out the solid core. Cut the leaves into thin shreds no more than 5 mm wide	For a large batch use a food processor. Possibly add some carrot or beetroot. You can add spices such as caraway or ginger but not too much as spices can kill the friendly fermenters. Green vegetables do not ferment well – I know; I have tried!
Put the shreds into a large plastic bowl that you can get your hands into	Do not use a metal container since the metal will contaminate the brew
Per 1 kg of cabbage plus other vegetable, add 20 g salt. Do weigh these ingredients until you get an eye for amounts	The salt multitasks by pulling water out of the cabbage (by osmosis), hardening pectins (a constituent of plant cell walls) for crunchiness, and inhibiting the growth of unfriendly bacteria (lactobacilli are more tolerant of salt) so the sauerkraut can be stored for longer periods of time

What to do	Notes
	Do not use Sunshine salt. The iodine it contains will kill the fermenting microbes. You will be relieved to hear this does not occur in the gut because iodine is rapidly absorbed from the upper gut
Get your hands in to massage the mix and dissolve the salt. Mix it uniformly throughout and feel the cabbage wilting. Carry on until the mix feels very wet	It is really important to make sure the salt is distributed uniformly otherwise the wrong microbes can flourish
Stuff it all into a jar as full as you can and press it down so the cabbage is covered with brine. Put on the lid but not too tightly as some gas is produced	I bought some sauerkraut online, then saved the jars for this job so you can do likewise OR use Kilner-type jars The cabbage shreds must be under the surface of the saline. If you can't achieve this, add some more salt water at the same concentration (20 g per 1 l water). Shreds which are not covered by liquid may allow oxygen-loving bacteria and yeasts to ferment to produce off flavours, scum and slime
Exclude as much air as you can by filling the jar as much as is possible, pack some bay leaves or horse-radish leaves on the top and pour a dollop of olive oil on the surface. This all helps to exclude oxygen	This is an anaerobic (oxygen-free) fermentation. Fermentation produces carbon dioxide which further helps exclude oxygen. The major microbe which ferments once oxygen has been used up is *Lactobacillus plantarum* – this is an excellent anti-inflammatory microbe and of proven benefit in inflammatory bowel disease. Do not stir a ferment or you will introduce oxygen and wreck it. In this event it may go brown, pink or produce a white film or slime
Put the lid on, but not too tight, OR get a special pot with an air lock	The ferment will produce gas; the lid must not be so tight that the pot explodes, but not so loose that oxygen can get in
The temperature for fermenting is important	18-22°C (65-72°F) is ideal – that means the highest shelf in my kitchen. Get a thermometer and measure this…it can be surprisingly warm

	Wait at least 4 weeks before tasting. Checking the taste too often introduces oxygen and you risk spoiling the batch. I have yet to have a jar explode. This is by contrast with my childhood experiments making ginger beer illicitly in the airing cupboard upstairs… Mother was cross because her clean linen was spoiled and Father was cross because his bucket of mealworms was contaminated*
Leave for at least 4, ideally 6, weeks	Then screw the lid on tight to prevent any oxygen getting in and refrigerate. This helps maintain the quality once you start to open and eat it

Kefir

Kefir does contain yeast, albeit a friendly one. Those who are yeast-allergic should avoid kefir. Instead, start with *Lactobacillus rhamnosus* culture. This microbe induces immune tolerance in the gut and helps switch off allergies.

l l long-life (i.e. sterile) coconut, hemp or soya milk
l dsp sugar

1. Pour the milk into a jug and stir in the sugar to give the kefir something to ferment.
2. Add a sachet of kefir (or use a previous ferment). Do place a lid on top but this does not need to be airtight; it will help to get the temperature high enough to ferment.
3. Keep in a warm place close to 37°C. You may need to use a yoghurt maker to achieve this. Within 18 hours it should have turned into a semi-solid, junket-like consistency, with some clear 'whey' on the surface. I drink this. If it is still sweet, allow it to ferment for longer until it tastes sharp.
4. Do not expect kefir to look like thick commercial yoghurt, but you can thicken it if preferred – see Lovely thick yoghurt below.

* **Note from Craig:** My father would have been delighted by such an enterprise. His favourite drink was a 'Gunner' – half ginger beer, half ginger ale with a dash of Angostura bitters (see https://en.wikipedia.org/wiki/Gunner_(cocktail))

5. Once fermented, keep the culture in the fridge, where it will ferment further but more slowly. This slower fermentation seems to improve the texture and flavour.
6. Once the jug is nearly empty, add another litre of PK milk and dsp sugar, stir it in, keep it at room temperature and away you go again. I don't even bother to wash up the jug – the slightly hard yellow bits on the edge I just stir in to restart the brew. This way a sachet of kefir lasts for life.

Added extras: Add a lump of creamed coconut to the ferment; this further feeds the kefir, imparts a delicious coconut flavour and thickens the culture.

I use a cup of kefir every day to swallow my daily supplements. This means at least one cupful is used daily and stops me forgetting about the culture lurking in my fridge. If you do forget, or leave it for a week on holiday, it may acquire a slightly pink membranous crust. Scrape this off and use what is underneath to get another batch going. I have tried eating this crust; it was a bit sharp on the palate but did me no harm!

Lovely thick yoghurt

500 ml kefir
½ cup coconut oil, warm and runny
½ tsp lecithin

1. Combine the fermented kefir, coconut oil and lecithin.
2. Whizz the mixture up in your Nutribullet, or equivalent.
3. Put it in the fridge and you will find it sets to a delicious gloop.[†]

Kvass

Kvass can be made from any fruit. It is a great way to consume fruit and all the good within, but without the sugar burden. It does require some yeast, so once again the

---

[†] **Footnote:** 'Gloop' is one of those words of unknown 20th century origin – anyone who has any idea how this word originated, please do contact us!

yeast-allergic must beware. It will also be very slightly alcoholic.

2 cups berries
I tsp honey or sugar (not necessary for sweeter berries such as strawberries or blueberries)
I tbsp whey from your kefir culture OR liquid from a previous culture

1. Add all the ingredients to a large glass Kilner-type jar with a wide mouth.
2. Fill it with warm water and cover with a lid to prevent oxygen getting in.
3. Leave in a warm room to ferment, ready to drink in 2-3 days, or when the sweetness has been replaced by sharpness.

We leave this chapter with the wise words of two famous chemists:

'I have wished to see chemistry applied to domestic objects…to fermentation….'
As Thomas Jefferson (1743 – 1826), American Founding Father and the principal author of the Declaration of Independence (1776), third President of the United States (1801-1809), wrote to Thomas Cooper (1759 –1839), an Anglo-American economist.[2] Cooper was described by Jefferson as 'one of the ablest men in America' and by John Adams as 'a learned ingenious scientific and talented madcap'.

'…and let me adde, that he that thoroughly understands the nature of Ferments and Fermentations, shall probably be much better able than he that Ignores them, to give a fair account of divers Phænomena of severall diseases (as well Feavers and others) which will perhaps be never thoroughly understood, without an insight into the doctrine of Fermentation.'

Robert Boyle FRS (25 January 1627 – 31 December 1691)[¶]

[¶] **Historical note:** Robert Boyle FRS (1627 – 1691) was an Anglo-Irish chemist, physicist and inventor. Today, Boyle is regarded as the first modern chemist. He is best known for three things: (1) Being an early instigator of the modern experimental 'scientific method'; (2) 'Boyle's Law', which shows the inverse proportionality between the absolute pressure and volume of a gas, within a closed system of constant temperature – namely, $PV = k$, where P is the pressure, V is the volume and k is some constant; (3) His book, *The Sceptical Chymist* (1661), which is seen as a cornerstone of modern chemistry (available at: www.gutenberg.org/cache/epub/22914/pg22914-images.html)

Chapter 19

PK water

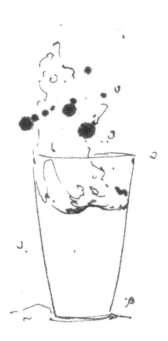

People eating Western diets are chronically dehydrated. Many realise this but the answer is not to drink more water. Indeed, some of the worst nourished patients I have ever seen are those who think it is healthy to drink several litres of water a day. Whilst one can drink pure water, one cannot pee pure water – urine always contains all the minerals. Such excessive consumption washes precious minerals out of the body and worsens the dehydration.

To understand what we need to do to hydrate the body properly, we need to return to elementary biology and remember osmosis.* This is the mechanism by which water is held within cells. The term 'Osmosis' describes this process:

> *'a process by which molecules of a solvent (ie water) tend to pass through a semipermeable membrane from a less concentrated solution into a more concentrated one*†

but the mechanism of such is explained by the fourth phase of water (see our book *The Energy Equation*). What this means is that for water to be held within a cell, firstly we need salts within that cell to 'pull' the water in; then we need fats to create a good (semipermeable) cell membrane.

This means that any water that is consumed must be balanced up with essential salts (a rounded teaspoonful daily of Sunshine salt; more if you exercise and sweat a lot) and an abundance of fats: saturated, unsaturated and essential fatty acids.

On the PK diet there are two vital types of fat in abundance. Firstly, there are the medium-chain fats which act primarily as fuels to power the body, from animals (lard), coconut or palm. Secondly, we need long-chain fats (which are liquid oils at room temperature) used primarily for making cell membranes. These oils (which include phospholipids) come from meat, eggs, vegetables, nuts, seeds and fish. Phospholipid oils have a water-loving end and a fat-loving end. They naturally line themselves up effort-lessly into a lipid sandwich with the water-loving end facing out and the fat-loving tails facing in. This is the basic structure of all cell membranes. Cholesterol is an essential part of these membranes.

---

* **Linguistic note:** 'Osmosis' derives from the Greek 'osmos', ὠσμός, 'a thrusting, a pushing,' from the stem of *othein* 'to thrust, to push'.

† **Scientific aside:** Many systems demonstrate the 'general idea' of osmosis – a kind of averaging out. In osmosis it is concentration levels that average out between liquids. A similar averaging out process happens with heat, as described by Newtonian cooling, where two bodies of different temperatures placed next to each other (this could be a warm body in a cool atmosphere) lose or gain heat in order to equalise the temperature of the system. Like many of his works, Newton published this result anonymously in 1701 in *Scala graduum Caloris. Calorum Descriptiones & signa*. Newton had his doubts about his abilities, and sometimes would check the response to a paper in the scientific community before announcing himself to be the author.

We have the sensation of thirst for good reason – it tells us how much to drink. I do not see any point in drinking over and above thirst requirements. Having said that, many drinks are diuretic – we should not be drinking them to quench thirst. Quench thirst with water – then use tea, herbal tea or coffee for pleasure and zip factor.

Ensuring good quality water

You should drink the best water you can – start with a good water filter.

We live in an increasingly polluted world. Furthermore, mains water is treated with chlorine, chlorine dioxide and, worse, chloramine. Whilst these are helpful in disinfecting water, they inevitably leave harmful residues and taste disgusting. Having become accustomed to spring water, my horses will not drink mains water. They will not eat a supermarket apple either. Water filters are an essential part of any PK kitchen and these are effective at removing chlorine and heavy metals.

However, if your water is fluoridated, a simple water filter won't do. They do not remove fluoride. Fluoride is a nasty toxic element ostensibly added to prevent tooth decay but really in order to dispose of a toxic by-product of industry. Fluoride is an endocrine (hormone) disruptor and may well part explain our current epidemic of hypothyroidism. It is also a probable carcinogen (bone cancer); it is deposited in and weakens bone (increasing fracture risk) and it readily combines with aluminium to encourage deposition of both in the brain, with dementia resulting. The current fashion for fluoride in water, dentistry and toothpaste is a health disaster.

No filter gets rid of fluoride completely; you will have to shop around to find one that suits. Many of the toxicities of fluoride result because iodine deficiency is pandemic, so using Sunshine salt will help protect against any residual fluoride.

Bottled water

If you are going to drink bottled water, use either glass or as large a plastic container as you can. Glass is inconvenient and heavy. However, for some of my patients who are very sensitive, water in glass bottles is the only water they can drink.

Most plastics contain softeners such as bisphenol A (BPA) which inevitably contaminate water. This explains the advice to avoid small bottles and also to not let them get warm. When left in heat, levels of BPA increase.[1] A large container reduces the surface area to volume ratio and so reduces contamination.

I am very fortunate to have several springs behind my house for water. If I were not so blessed, then for drinking and cooking purposes I would install a rainwater harvesting system and use an ultraviolet light to disinfect it.

I also love sparkling water. Consider purchasing a soda stream for carbonated water.

Conclusion

Craig leaves you with a quotation that was ancient even during the time of Pliny the Elder (died 79 AD), who himself quoted it. The fact that the first half of this quote is the most remembered perhaps reflects on the nature of mankind itself:

In vino veritas, in aqua sanitas.
In wine there is truth, in water there is health.

But make sure it is the right kind of aqua!
Sarah Myhill

Chapter 20

Feasting and alcohol

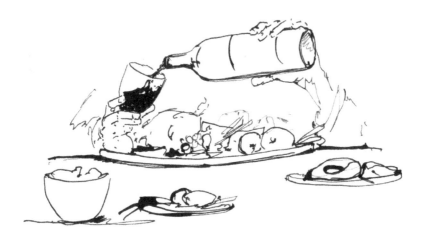

Primitive man feasted and drank alcohol and so shall I. Doing both is sociable and fun. Alcohol has a disinhibiting effect, so we socialise more easily. My jokes are so much improved by a glass of cider. The enjoyment of gathering is enhanced by good food and booze. Enjoyment is good for us and laughter is the best medicine.

> *The art of medicine consists of amusing the patient while Nature cures the disease.*
> Voltaire, 1694 – 1778

> *If you wish to glimpse inside a human soul and get to know the man, don't bother analyzing his ways of being silent, of talking, of weeping, or seeing how much he is moved by noble ideas; you'll get better results if you just watch him laugh. If he laughs well, he's a good man... All I claim to know is that laughter is the most reliable gauge of human nature.*
>
> Fyodor Dostoyevsky, 1821 – 1881

The key to feasting* and alcohol is to do both occasionally and not to excess. My definition of that is once a week at home, for any social event[†] and most days when on holiday.

Once established, PK taste buds change and high-sugar junk foods become unpalatable. Alcohol is a general anaesthetic the stages of which are (modified from *Gaddum's Pharmacology* 1950):

Dizzy and delightful. Amnesia and analgesia[†]

Drunk and disorderly. Uninhibited response to stimuli

Dead drunk. Surgical anaesthesia

Dangerously deep. Vital centre depression

Dead.

---

* **Historical note:** A famous feast took place at Brighton Royal Pavilion on 18 January 1817. It was given by the Prince Regent (later George IV) and included over 100 dishes, was prepared by 'celebrity' chef Antonin Careme, and was designed to impress the Grand Duke Nicolas of Russia. The dishes included: the head of a great sturgeon in champagne; jellied partridge with mayonnaise; pigeons in crayfish butter; terrine of larks; rose ice cream; the Royal Pavilion rendered in pastry. You can buy an A2-size copy of the menu at the Royal Pavilion today. See: https://brightonmuseums.org.uk/shop/product/caremes-menu-poster/

[†] Craig is alcohol-intolerant, but he can still feast, and much amusement can be had watching good friends get to the 'dizzy and delightful' stage.

Stop drinking at the dizzy and delightful stage (for me that is one pint of cider).

After a jolly, get back on the wagon. If you are unable to, then you have switched on a serious addiction for which complete abstinence is the only safe course. Remember alcohol is a good servant but a bad master.

> 'Squiffy, have you ever felt a sort of strange emptiness in the heart? A sort of aching void of the soul?'
> 'Oh, rather!'
> 'What do you do about it?'
> 'I generally take a couple of cocktails.'
>
> P.G. Wodehouse, 1881 – 1975, *Doctor Sally*

Chapter 21

Vegetarians and vegans

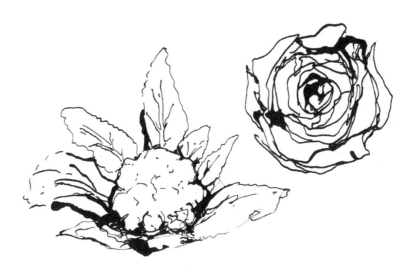

I like many have deep concerns for animal welfare. I am so fortunate to be able to rear my own pigs, obtain eggs from my own chickens and ducks and purchase lamb and beef locally, all of which I know is free range and grass fed. I encourage all my vegetarians and vegans to move to consuming organic eggs, organic butter and perhaps organic meat as these animals are well cared for. In my area of expertise – namely, chronic fatigue syndrome and ME – I know that the vegetarians and vegans are at a high risk of these conditions compared with omnivores. The nutritional concerns are that vegan (and vegetarian without dairy) diets tend to have the problems listed in Table 16.1.

Table 16.1: Problems with vegetarian and vegan (Vs) diets

Issue	Why this is problematic	Actions
High in carbohydrates	This is a risk for upper fermenting gut and all the problems that accompany such	See Chapter 3
High in fruit	Fruit contains the dangerous fruit sugar fructose	See Chapter 33
Low in protein	This is a risk for weight gain through protein leverage (hunger not satisfied)	See Chapter 3
Low in fat	Fat is essential for all cells membranes	See Chapter 3
	Without fat there is poor absorption of fat-soluble vitamins (A, D, E and K)	See Chapter 3
Lacking in specific amino acids	Only animal protein has the full spectrum of amino acids that humans require	The Vs must do a tricky balancing act to get all the essentials
Lacking in the omega-3 essential fatty acids (EFAs)	Most plant, seed and nut oils are so high in omega 6 EFAs there is a serious imbalance; there should be 4:1 of omega 6 to omega 3.	
	Even if there is sufficient omega 3, many people cannot make the essential fatty acids EPA and DHA downstream (naturally present in fish oil)	See Chapter 3
Lacking in vitamin B12	Vitamin B12 is found only in animal products; it is particularly high in shellfish and offal	All Vs need to supplement this
Low in creatine	Creatine is an essential raw material for energy production	All Vs need to supplement this
Low in carnitine	Carnitine is an essential peptide for delivering fuel to mitochondria	All Vs need to supplement this
Low in vitamin A	To get enough vitamin A you have to consume a lot of squash and carrots and be able to convert the carotene they contain to vitamin A	All Vs need to supplement this

Low in raw materials for connective tissue	Bone broth is a rich source of nutrients to build strong connective tissue	See Chapter 12
High in vegetables	This is a mixed blessing – the plant toxins require excellent liver function to deal with them and include toxins from legumes (lectins, tannins and phytic acid), quinoa (tannins, phytic acid, saponins), kale and other cruciferous greens (oxalates, goitrogens), nuts (phytic acid, tannins), rice (arsenic), wheat and corn (lectins, gluten, mycotoxins, phytic acid), soya (lectins) and potatoes and tomatoes (lectins)	Ensure good energy delivery mechanisms and supplements to support the liver's detoxification mechanisms
High in soya	Soya is often genetically modified, is pro-inflammatory, a phyto-oestrogen (feminising effect), often mould-contaminated, and is high in lectins	Avoid, except for fermented products and soya milk
Include unnatural foods	Quorn is an example of such. The jury is still out but I am instinctively suspicious	Avoid

Simply introducing eggs and butter (allergy permitting) into the diet would obviate many of the above problems.

Anyone considering a vegan PK diet must consider all the above issues, balance up their diet, take the necessary supplements and stick to those for life. Even then I cannot guarantee that they will be as healthy as my PK omnivores.

Chapter 22

The carnivore diet

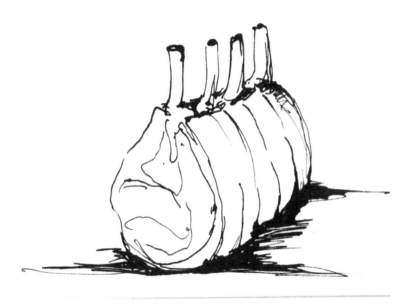

There are three common dietary starting points to treat disease. For most, the PK diet is both start and finish, but with more serious disease, especially gut pathology, the starting point may be the carnivore diet or fasting (see Chapter 23). The reasons for the carnivore diet are:

1. Low allergen. It is unusual to be allergic to meat. Meats are the least toxic foods we can eat. Look at life from the point of view of a plant – it does not want to be eaten so it makes itself as poisonous as it can, as described in Chapters 16 and 21. Animals can run away to avoid being eaten and so don't 'need' to be toxic. (Here we are talking about organic, non-factory-farmed meats. Do the best you can to obtain the best quality meat you can and try to avoid meat that has had preservatives added, or that has formerly had its growth enhanced by the use of antibiotics.)

2. Meats are very low in carbohydrate so there is little potential for fermentation in the gut.
3. Meats are energy-dense and smaller meals are more easily dealt with by the gut.
4. The enzymes for its digestion are contained within meat and so, again, more easily dealt with by the gut. (If you are in any doubt here, compare the size of a carnivorous gut, like a dog's, with a vegetarian gut, like a cow's).
5. Meats are rich in nutrients for healing. It is likely that most Westerners (who are not doing the PK diet!) have gut damage and meat contains all the raw materials for repair work.
6. Meat is a complete food. There is everything within one animal to nourish another animal.

The first scientific study that used the carnivore diet was published in 1930 (McClellan and Du Bois). Vilhjalmur Stefansson, an anthropologist and Arctic traveller, was convinced that the Arctic Inuit people's fat- and meat-based diet was nutritionally complete and healthy. To prove this, he and a fellow-traveller took part in a year-long study where they ate only animal fat and meat, without vitamin or mineral supplements. At the end of the year there were no signs of vitamin deficiencies or kidney problems in Stefansson or his companion; they did not suffer fatigue, they were mentally alert and physically active, and showed no specific physical changes in any system of the body.[1]

What is the carnivore diet?

Drinks
Water, flat or fizzy, with vitamin C
Black tea and coffee (away from mealtimes)
Bone broth as below – with a pinch of Sunshine salt this is remarkably satisfying

Meals
At first all should be meat only
If you are sure you are not allergic to, add in fish
If you are sure you are not allergic to, add in eggs

Extras

Take your usual nutritional supplements including 5 g Sunshine salt per day

- You need to do this diet for at least 2 weeks. This allows time for healing and repair and for diet, die-off and detox (DDD) reactions (see Chapter 5).
- If you are not sure, stick with the diet for longer. In Dr John Mansfield's arthritis study some patients took six weeks to respond.[2, 3]
- Once improved, reintroduce foods one at a time (to check for allergic reactions).
- Reintroduce probiotic foods early, especially sauerkraut (see Chapter 18).
- The end point should be the PK diet.

Bone broth

Bone broth made from boiled bones is an essential part of any PK kitchen. It formed a vital part of any Mediaeval kitchen and is detailed in Mrs Beeton's famous *Book of Household Management*.* It imparts fabulous flavour and texture to soups and stews and makes for a delicious hot drink. Once addiction is out of the equation, we acquire a taste for those things which are good for our health (see Chapter 15: Human pharmacognosy). This makes perfect evolutionary sense and encourages us to seek out nutritious foods of which bone broth is a vital one.

> Any bones – raw or leftovers, meat, fish, chicken
> Pig's head
> Tough offcuts of meat – oxtail, neck of lamb, pig's trotters, calf's foot, the sinewy bits of the heart, diaphragm
> Water – which may be from cooked vegetables but must be good quality (see Chapter 19: PK water).

---

* Mrs Beeton's *Book of Household Management* when first published in 1861 consisted of 1112 pages and contained over 900 recipes. Isabella Mary Beeton (née Mayson; 1836 –1865; died age 28 from infection after the birth of her fourth child) said of it subsequently: 'I must frankly own, that if I had known, beforehand, that this book would have cost me the labour which it has, I should never have been courageous enough to commence it.'

1. You need a slow-cooker.
2. Chop up the bones so the bone marrow can leach out.
3. Allow the bones to simmer gently in the water for hours or days.
4. Whenever needed for a hot drink, soup or stews, ladle out the broth and add a sprinkling of Sunshine salt for extra flavour.
5. Every few days, allow the whole pot to cool, lift off the fat for cooking, pour off the stock for keeping, use the denuded bones in the garden as a fertiliser, and start another brew.

Shakespeare has other suggestions for bone broth ingredients which, as you can see, are all PK. He was a clever boy and clearly knew what was good for him…:

Double, double toil and trouble;
Fire burn and caldron bubble.
Fillet of a fenny snake,
In the caldron boil and bake;
Eye of newt and toe of frog,
Wool of bat and tongue of dog,
Adder's fork and blind-worm's sting,
Lizard's leg and howlet's wing,
For a charm of powerful trouble,
Like a hell-broth boil and bubble.
        From *Macbeth*, 'The Song of The Witches', William Shakespeare (1564 – 1616)

Rillette

I make this from my pig heads and trotters. It is important to include the eyes because anything made from such will see you through the week… boom boom! (Craig)

1. Boil up the heads and trotters until the coverings are soft, then allow to cool.
2. Use your hands to separate the meat, lard, fat, brains, tongue and connective tissue from the skin and bones.
3. Put these pickings, slightly warm, into your Nutribullet/equivalent with Sunshine salt and pepper and whizz up into a gloop.

4. Put into pots then into the fridge – it then sets to a firm consistency.
5. Use like paté.
6. The remaining skin and bones can go back into the stock pot.
7. You will be left with hands covered with fat. Rub this into your skin — lard is the perfect fat for skin.[†]

Rosemary Segrott's brawn

Make this as for rillette but include beef shin – this imparts a lovely meaty texture.

Bacon-wrapped liver pieces

Liver – the fresher the better
Bacon

1. Cut the liver into small pieces.
2. Wrap each piece in a thin slice of bacon.
3. Put the bacon-wrapped liver pieces onto a greased baking sheet and bake at 200°C for 10 minutes while covered with a lid.
4. Then fry the pieces uncovered.
5. Add salt only when about to serve.

[†] Sheep shearers know lard is perfect for the skin too: after a day's shearing the callused hands and arms of these tough farmers become as soft as the proverbial baby's bottom. This derives from the waterproofing lard, lanolin. Indeed 'wool fat soap' was a very common traditional soap, made from lanolin. Modern versions of such contain many additives for colour and 'fragrance' and are poor cousins to the original.

Offal – the best ways to cook it

Following a successful hunt, the carcass would have been shared out by primitive man. Top brass received the offal. Second class citizens, often women, got the muscle meat. Offal is the most nutritious foods.‡ The most nutritious is also the most delicious. We Westerners have forgotten the value of offal. Because offal is so rich in enzymes, it 'rots' within hours and this changes the flavours to 'off'. Offal must be cooked as fresh as is possible!

Liver and kidney from beef, pork, lamb, chicken, duck, goose

Do not overcook or it goes tough. Flash fry so the centre remains pink. Divine!

Heart from beef, pork, lamb:

Cut off the white, tough arteries and veins and lob into the stock pot.

Slice thinly. Again, flash fry so it remains pink in the middle. This is a treat that I love to share with my Patterdale terrier Nancy because even greedy me cannot eat a whole heart.

Mr Leopold Bloom ate with relish the inner organs of beasts and fowls. He liked thick giblet soup, nutty gizzards, a stuffed roast heart, liver slices fried with crust crumbs, fried hencods' roes.

James Joyce, 1882 - 1941, Ulysses

‡ **Classical aside:** Not only in fiction does offal have a pedigree. A much favoured dish during the time of the Roman Empire was the 'shield of Minerva', which was composed of pike liver, the brains of pheasant and peacock, and flamingo tongues. The name the Shield of Minerva relates to the Medusa story; Medusa, a beautiful woman and priestess of the Goddess Minerva, was caught kissing the God Neptune in a temple dedicated to Minerva. Minerva was incensed by this, and so turned Medusa into a monster, replacing her hair with hissing snakes. As further punishment, Medusa turned any living creature she looked upon into stone. Perseus managed to avoid this petrification because when he approached Medusa, he used the Shield of Minerva to see her reflection, thus avoiding eye contact and with that, he was able to behead her.

Pork meatballs

This recipe works equally well for lamb and beef. With chicken, use more fat.

> 500 g minced meat (pork leg)
> If you can get brain, that makes for a delicious addition to the mix
> 4 tbsp fat
> 2 eggs
> Sunshine salt

1. Preheat your oven to 200°C.
2. Mix all the ingredients together and form into golf-ball size meatballs.
3. Bake in the overn for 40 minutes.

Michelle McCullagh's liver pancakes

These are super-easy and deliciously nutritious and versatile. They are a great way of using up a glut of eggs – I make large batches and freeze the pancakes to get out another time. This is a much healthier way to celebrate Pancake Day than the usual.

> raw liver (any kind – pig, lamb, pheasant, duck, cow, whatever)
> eggs (approx. 1/3 quantity of liver)
> I large dollop animal fat or coconut oil

1. Put the liver and eggs in your Nutribullet/equivalent and whiz until totally blended – it should be a beautiful dark pink colour. (It doesn't really matter how many eggs; the more you put in the fluffier your pancakes will be, the less the more livery.)
2. Add the animal fat or coconut oil to a frying pan and put this on a high heat.
3. Once sizzling, take spoonfuls of the mixture from your Nutribullet into the frying pan, to make several small pancakes. They will cook very quickly and as soon as they are stiff enough to flip, do so and cook the other side.
4. Serve hot with a fried breakfast, or at lunch time with a bowl of spinach soup or cold as a starter with butter on.

Nest-eggs

100 g (a handful) minced meat (beef, lamb, pork, chicken)
Sunshine salt
1 egg
Slice of bacon

1. Preheat your oven to 200°C.
2. Fashion the meat into a doughnut shape (with a hole in the middle) and place on a baking tray.
3. Crack a whole egg into the hollow and cover it with a slice of bacon.
4. Bake in the oven for 40 minutes.

Beefsteak or venison tartare

The least cooking, the more nutritious. Arguably raw is the best way to eat meat. Once you are past the 'yuck' factor, this is delicious. 'Chewing meat', raw, was a treat my mother occasionally lobbed off the table at me when she was preparing a beef stew. Yum yum!

500 g minced steak (must be a tender cut)
2 egg yolks
Fat
Sunshine salt

1. Mince the meat.
2. Mix it with the egg yolks, fat and salt.
3. Put the mixture into the refrigerator for one day to be aged before serving.

Chapter 23

Fasting
– a great therapeutic tool

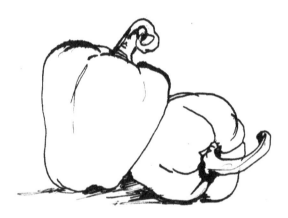

Primitive man feasted and fasted. So do all carnivores. It makes perfect evolutionary sense that to fast enhances physical and mental performance – it made Man a better hunter. He got hungry for food… and we use this very word to describe the will and energy to succeed. Mozart produced his finest works when hungry for money, as did Van Gogh and Dickens. Being hungry enhances performance.

Fasting is the first principle of medicine: fast and see the strength of the spirit reveal itself.

Rumi, 1207 – 1273, Persian poet, faqih, Islamic scholar, theologian, and Sufi mystic originally from Greater Khorasan in Greater Iran

Why fasting is such a great tool

Fasting has these benefits:

1. **Helps weight loss** – see Chapter 24.
2. **Reduces hypertension (high blood pressure) and high cholesterol (hyper-cholestrolaemia)** – Both of course normalise on a PK diet. Fasting makes this happen more quickly. If they do not normalise, look for other causes such as high homocysteine, thyroid problems and sleep disturbance.
3. **Restores insulin sensitivity** – Insulin resistance is the hallmark of type 2 diabetes. If not already in ketosis, fasting empties glycogen stores, reverses insulin resistance and is the most direct way to lose weight and to reverse metabolic syndrome and diabetes. Diabetics and their doctors are often anxious about blood sugar dropping dangerously low. This can *only* happen if the diabetic is taking prescribed medication to lower their blood sugar. The key is to monitor blood sugar levels closely and as they come down, as they inevitably will, reduce the dose of medication. Type 2 diabetics should be able to stop all medication. Type 1 diabetics *must* use continuous blood sugar monitoring such as Dexcom. They eventually need a much smaller dose of insulin. Remember Dr Ian Lake, the type 1 diabetic in Chapter 4 (page 51) who fasted for five days whilst running 100 miles? He was running on fats and his blood sugars remained absolutely stable throughout. In this way the 'brittle' diabetics are stabilised. Doctors always fret about their patients being in ketosis because the only state they know about is diabetic ketoacidosis – a dire emergency that occurs when blood sugar is very high. This problem is entirely preventable with careful blood sugar monitoring. (Please note that if you are taking bowel tolerance doses of vitamin C this will give false highs on home-testing blood sugar kits which rely on glucose oxidase. I have to say this gave me a terrible fright when I tested my own blood sugar to find it at 7.8 mmol/l (reference range 4.5 – 5.6 mmol/l). I sent off the same sample to the lab which came back at 5.4 mmol/l. Phew!) (Please see our book *Prevent and Cure Diabetes* for more detail.)
4. **Builds muscle and improves fitness** – Human growth hormone spikes with fasting; this results in more muscle being laid down (so we can run faster and throw those primitive spears further) together with fat burning. Metabolic rate increases by up to 14%. Again, we see that fasting enhances performance – the

Samurai warrior fasted before fighting. Indeed, before battle, he was advised to drink only: 'hot water that had been poured over rice' (*The Hundred Rules of War*, Tsukahara Bokuden, 1489 – 1571).

5. **Helps to treat infections** – All infections, including viral ones, are fed by sugar. Fasting and rest mean all energy is available for the immune system to fight the good fight.

Fast a cold, fast a fever.

Old adage
[Myhill adapted, with apologies]

6. **Aids detoxification** – The greatest source of toxic stress in the body comes from the gut (see Chapter 2: What is the PK diet?). Obviously fasting greatly reduces this burden. Fat is a repository for fat-soluble toxins (see Chapter 5: Trouble shooting – DDD reactions).
7. **Promotes autophagy ('self-eating')** – When fuel and raw materials do not come through from the gut, the body looks to the self for such. Unlike carbs and fat, protein cannot be stored in the body for later use. During a fast, the body obtains protein from recycling old, worn out cells and this is called autophagy. This is the metabolic equivalent of spring cleaning and it has profound beneficial effects. Autophagy has profound anti-inflammatory, rejuvenating, anti-cancer and healing properties. Indeed, for thousands of years fasting has been used to treat an alphabet of disease: arterial disease and arthritis, brain tumours, cancer, dementia, epilepsy, fatigue, hypertension, gastritis, Hodgkin's and more.

Fasting is the greatest remedy – the physician within.
Paracelsus, 15th century Swiss German Renaissance physician and botanist

8. **Shifts stem cells from a dormant state to a state of self-renewal** so it is good for:
    *   the immune system – old cells are killed off and young front-line fighters grown.
    *   the brain – neurones make more connections.
    *   the rest of the body – new young cells for the gut, liver, skin, blood vessels, connective tissue, heart, muscle and bone.
9. **Helps to treat cancer** – We know the ketogenic diet starves cancer cells of

sugar, without which they cannot be fuelled. Fasting increases ketosis even more – combine the PK diet with the immune stimulation of fasting and vitamin C to bowel tolerance and, yes, you are really winning! Autophagy digests cancer cells too and we know fasting before and during chemotherapy enhances the effects of, and minimises the side effects of, treatment. Fasting also enhances the effect of radiotherapy. I would recommend fasting on the day before and the day of such treatments, possibly longer.

10. **Helps to treat dementia** – Consultant neurologist Dr Dale Bredesen cured dementia with a ketogenic diet. Fasting does this faster. Remember, foggy brain is an early symptom of dementia.[1]

How to go about fasting

First get keto-adapted. This avoids many of the diet, die-off and detox (DDD) reactions (see Chapter 5) which are an inevitable result of getting into ketosis. Anticipate:

- Social opprobrium: When I announced I was going to do a five-day fast my friends were immediately anxious for my physical and mental health!
- Fear of hunger and, accompanying such, fear of fatigue and of foggy brain. As you will discover, there is nothing to fear and, with time and practice, you will look forward to your fasts. Hunger is greatly ameliorated by telling your brain that you are going to do it regardless of its nagging. You make your mind up and feel proud that you can do what all others fear.

In the afternoon, the digestion of the meal deprives me of the incomparable lightness which characterizes the fast days.
Adalbert De Vogue, 1924 – 2011, Benedictine monk

I fast for greater physical and mental efficiency.
Plato, 424/423 – 348/347 BC, who was taught by Socrates and who taught Aristotle

What you can consume

- Yes, you must drink water and take electrolytes. The ideal mix is spring water with Sunshine salt. I add a squeeze of fresh lemon.

- Clear liquids such as black tea, black coffee, green tea.
- Bone broth with a sprinkling of Sunshine salt.
- Carry on your usual nutritional supplements including vitamin C, at least 5 grams or to bowel tolerance.

If you are on prescription medication, carry on but monitor the effects. The need for most comes down, especially drugs for hypertension (check blood pressure daily), diabetes (monitor blood sugar), asthma (check peak flow), painkillers, anti-inflammatories and, I suspect, thyroid hormones.

Do not confuse hunger pangs with greed or need. Use hot water, lemon juice and bone broth to postpone the 'breakthrough' waves of hunger, and by the time you are sipping you will find that the wave has passed.

How long to fast

Start by eating all your PK meals within a 10-hour window of time. This means you are fasting 14 hours a day. This is a great start.

Then move to one day a week of a 24-hour fast. This means you simply skip one breakfast a week, assuming you are eating breakfast and supper only on a PK diet. This is where you should be before starting a fast. If you are already PK, autophagy cuts in at 16 hours.

Do a two-day fast once a month. This means you skip two breakfasts and one evening meal.

Perhaps fast more depending on whatever health problems you have.

Conclusion

I am greedy and love food. I reckon fasting gives me the best of both worlds – I can be greedy (without bingeing) on feast days and not be hungry, helpless or hapless on fasting days. When I fast the usual chores of shopping, cooking, washing up and clearing away vanish. I have more time and energy for all else. I have now come to joyfully anticipate my fasts.

Fasting is the most inexpensive therapeutic tool, it multitasks as above and the potential for side-effects or harm is miniscule. I like that sort of medicine.

Chapter 24

Easy weight loss with the PK diet

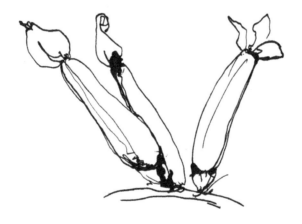

We know calorie restriction does not work. It is easy to see why. The prolonged mild starvation of reducing calories makes the body believe there is a famine. It moves into survival mode with the body shutting down energy expenditure. The usual clinical picture is that yes, weight is lost for the first week or so, but then the body adjusts by matching energy expenditure to energy delivery. The low energy expenditure results in physical fatigue, mental fatigue and depression. Weight loss ceases which adds to the misery. That poor, half-starved mortal remains fat, fatigued, foggy and in a funk hole. The answer is to take advantage of the inherent, metabolic inertia in the body that means it takes several days for metabolism to slow (see Chapter 23) and practise intermittent fasting as follows:

Step 1 – Get PK adapted.

Step 2 – Calculate the calories you should need for normal energetic life (see Chapter 3).

Step 3 – *Eat* these calories for five days of the week. Do not eat less than this amount or you will switch off calorie burning and go into starvation mode.

Step 4 – For two days in every week (consecutive or separate) either fast or substantially reduce your calories. Throughout these two days, you will continue to burn fat at your normal rate. Mental and physical energy will remain normal, but your weekly calorie consumption will be reduced by at least two sevenths (28%).

Step 5 – If this system (known as the '5:2 diet') fails, then get your thyroid checked (see our book *Ecological Medicine*, Chapter 13).

The How in more detail

Take a look at Figure 24.1. This supposes that your calculated 'normal energetic' calorie intake is 2000 kcal and that you have decided to reduce this to 500 kcal on the two fasting days you have chosen. (Many people infact find it easier to fast for two consecutive days – the second day is often easier and you will be in autophagy for longer.)

Figure 24.1 shows how, when you reduce calorie intake in this way, the calorie burn remains at 2000 kcal per day throughout the week, meaning that on the two fasting days, 3000 kcal of weight are lost. Altogether, 1 lb (0.45 kg) of body fat contains between about 3436 and 3752 calories (kcal). If instead you fasted for two days, as opposed to reducing daily calorie intake to 500 kcal, you would lose 4000 kcal – that is, well over 1 lb (half a kilo) of fat a week – great progress.

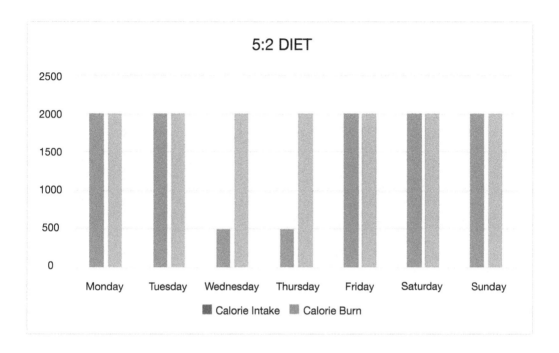

Figure 24.1: The effect of a 5:2 diet on calorie burn

If, however, you took the 'prolonged starvation' route, you can see from Figure 24.2 that there might be weight loss initially but that, as your body switched into survival mode, then calorie burn would reduce to equalise with calorie intake and no further weight loss would occur. In other words, the 5:2 approach takes advantage of metabolic inertia while prolonged calorie restriction gives time for metabolic adjustment.

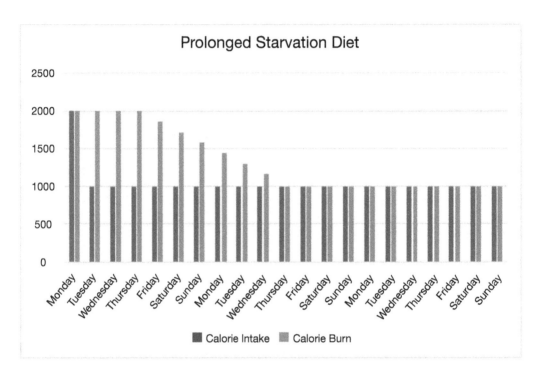

Figure 24.2: The effects of prolonged calorie restriction on calorie burn

The modern fad to treat obesity is bariatric surgery (252,000 operations in the USA in 2018[1]). Yes, it works for weight loss, but health losses include: dumping syndrome, malnutrition, vomiting, ulcers, bowel obstruction, hernia, blood clots, gallstones and more. Intermittent fasting is more effective and a darn sight safer.

Appendices

Appendix 1

The carbohydrate content of common foods

This appendix consists of lists of the carbohydrate content of vegetables and salads, fruits and berries, and nuts and seeds. It is far from exhaustive. The carbohydrate values are for the most part taken from the USDA (United States Department of Agriculture) database entry. This online database is not user-friendly. The best way to navigate it is to use the Google search engine and type in the name of the food followed by 'carbs'. Expect to see the box below pop up on the right side of your screen based on the most current USDA figures – the example is for 'Brussels sprouts'. This may not work with all search engines.

Total carbohydrate is a measure of sugars, starch and fibre. We are interested in net carbs (sugars and starch, with fibre excluded) because these provide a sugar load and may be fermented by unfriendly upper-gut microbes. By contrast, fibre is fermented within the lower gut by friendly microbes into short chain fatty acids, which are highly desirable. In the example in Figure A1.1 we have 9 grams (g) of total carbohydrate of which 3.8 g is fibre leaving 5.2 g of starch and sugar per 100 g of Brussels sprouts.

I have separated carbohydrates into:

- **green categories:** (up to 5 g/100 g or <5% carb) which you can eat pretty much ad lib (or you would have to eat over 500 g to start to run into problems. Even greedy me can't manage that).
- **amber:** (5-10 g/100 g or >5% carb but <10%); you will need to measure these out carefully.
- **red:** (10-13 g per 100 g or >10% carb but < 13%) which you will need to ration carefully; they will tend to switch on addictive eating. Occasional use only as it is easy to eat too much.

Nutrition Facts

Brussels sprouts

Sources include: USDA

Amount Per 100 grams

Calories 43

	% Daily Value*
Total Fat 0.3 g	0%
Saturated fat 0.1 g	0%
Cholesterol 0 mg	0%
Sodium 25 mg	1%
Potassium 389 mg	11%
Total Carbohydrate 9 g	3%
Dietary fiber 3.8 g	15%
Sugar 2.2 g	
Protein 3.4 g	6%

Figure A1.1: An example of the USDA database of food values – Brussels sprouts

- **high-carb foods:** (>13 g per 100 g or >13% carb); these are highly addictive and should be used with extreme caution.

You may, of course, find differing carbohydrate values online or in various versions of the products listed. As we have said, we can teach you the rules of the game – it is up to you how you play it. These Tables, then, are guidelines and if you find, for example, a less 'carby' chocolate, then good for you! (Craig hates the stuff (chocolate) and always has, and so doesn't have this problem.) You could argue similarly for most food types. While the figures in the Tables are taken mostly from the USDA, there is much disagreement. The point is that we are trying to give you guidelines and cannot account for every single variation.

Table A1.1: Green foods (<5% carb)

Vegetables	Salads	Nuts, nut butters and seeds	Fruits for pudding	Grains and pulses	Miscellaneous
Chicory 0.7 Pak choi 1.2 Curly kale 1.3 Spinach 1.4 Asparagus 1.8 Collard greens 2.0 Marrow 2.0 Courgette (zucchini) 2.1 Swiss chard 2.1 Mushrooms 2.3 Bamboo shoots 2.8 Aubergine (eggplant) 3.0 Cauliflower 3.0 Cabbage 3.5 Green beans 3.6 Okra 3.8 Fennel 3.9 Turnip 4.2 Broccoli 4.4 Spring onions 4.4 Cress 4.9	Alfalfa sprouts 0.2 Endive 0.3 Watercress 0.8 Celery 1.4 Lettuce, romaine 1.2 Lettuce 1.6 Radishes 1.8 Chives 2 Avocado 2 Tomatoes* 2.7* Olives 3.8 Cucumber 3.1	Hemp seeds 2.8 Brazil nuts 4.0 Pecans 4.0	Rhubarb 2.7	Linseeds (aka Flax seeds) 2.0 (which is why the PK bread is so good!)	Vinegars 0 Sunflower lecithin 0 Soy sauce 4.1

* **Dinner party conversation note:** Tomato – fruit or vegetable? The key question is, does 'it' have seeds? If yes, then technically it is a fruit. So, the tomato is a fruit, along with cucumbers, squash, green beans and pumpkins. We also eat leaves (lettuces), stems (celery), roots (carrots) and flowers (broccoli). The confusion about 'fruit' and 'vegetable' arises because of the difference in what a scientist calls a fruit and what a cook calls a fruit. True fruits are developed from the ovary in the base of the flower, and contain the seeds of the plant. However, cultivated forms may be seedless. Blueberries, raspberries and oranges are types of fruit, and so are many kinds of nut. Some plants have a soft part which supports the seeds and these are also called a 'fruit', even though they are not developed from the ovary: the strawberry is an example. Cooks generally call things vegetables when they are used in savoury rather than sweet cooking. Occasionally the term 'fruit' may be used to refer to

Table A1.2: Amber foods (5-10% carb)

Vegetables	Salads	Nuts, nut butters and seeds	Fruits for pudding	Grains and pulses	Miscellaneous
Brussels sprouts 5.2 Squash, spaghetti 5.5 Artichoke (globe) 6.0 Pumpkin 6.5 Corn, baby sweetcorn 6.5 Swede 6.7 Celeriac 7.2 Beetroot 7.2 Carrots 7.2 Onions 7.3 Squash, butternut 10.0	Capsicum pepper 7.5	Coconut 6.0 Macadamia nuts 6.0 Walnuts 7.0 Peanuts 7.0 Hazelnuts 7.0 Chia seeds 8.0 Poppy seeds 8.0 Tiger nuts 9.0 Pine nuts 9.3 Almonds 10.0	Raspberry 5.0 Blackberry 5.0 Gooseberry 5.7 Strawberry 6.0 Lemon 6.2 Cranberry 6.4 Black/redcurrant 6.6 Cantaloupe 7.2 Water melon 7.6 Lime 8.2 Mulberry 8.3 Peach 8.5 Apricot 9.0 Nectarine 9.3 Grapefruit 9.4 Plum 9.6 Orange 9.6	Peas 9.0	Hummus 8.0

a part of a plant which is not a fruit, but which is used in sweet cooking: rhubarb, for example. As this is in part a cookbook, foods have been categorised as the mood takes. Going back to the original question, the answer is that a tomato is technically the fruit of the tomato plant, but that it's used as a vegetable in cooking. However, if you want to be a smarty pants, you could go on and say that, although technically a fruit, tomatoes have been classified as vegetables according to the US Supreme Court. In 1893, there was a 'tomato ruling' in a case brought by the Nix family against Edward Hedden, collector at the Port of New York, to recover fees they spent transporting tomatoes. The Nixes sued under the Tariff of 1883, which required taxes on imported vegetables — but not on fruit. So the Nixes lost…

Table A1.3: Red foods (>10% carb)

Vegetables	Salads	Nuts, nut butters and seeds	Fruits for pudding	Grains and pulses	Miscellaneous
Leeks 12 Lentils 12		Sesame seeds 11.0 Sunflower seeds 11.0 Psyllium husks 11.1 Tahini seeds 11.5 Pumpkin seed butter 12.0 Coriander seeds 12.0 Caraway seeds 12.0	Clementine 10.3 Cherry 10.4 Elderberry 11.0 Guava 11.0 Satsuma 11.2 Blueberry 11.3 Apple 11.3 Pineapple 11.6 Pear 11.9 Kiwi 12.0	Oats 10.3	100% dark chocolate – 14.0 (depending on the brand and its cocoa fat content)

Table A1.4: High-carb foods (>13%)

Vegetables	Salads	Nuts, nut butters and seeds	Fruits for pudding	Grains and pulses	Miscellaneous
Parsnip 13.1 Shallots 13.8 Potatoes 14.8 Artichokes (Jerusalem) 15 Sweet potato 28.0		Peanut butter 14.0 Chestnut butter 16.5 Almond nut butter 17.5 Pistachios 18.0 Pomegranate seeds 18.7 Chestnuts 26.0 Cashews 26.7 Cumin seeds 35.0 Pumpkin seeds 36.0 Hazelnut butter 57.0	Passionfruit 13.0 Quince 13.1 Mango 13.4 Pomegranate 15.0 Grapes 16.1 Banana 20.4	Quinoa 17 Brown rice 21 Kidney beans 35 Haricot beans (as in baked beans) 36 White rice up to 82% (My most hated breakfast cereals, which must be nameless, are 89% carb)	Cacao powder 16.5 85% dark chocolate 22.5 Carob 23.5 Cocoa powder 25.0

You can eat anything – it is a question of how much. You can consume large amounts of low-carb, small amounts of high-carb and judge whether you have the balance right through testing for ketones (see Chapter 4).

Zero-carb foods

All the following can be eaten ad lib as they are zero carb:
• All fats and oils

Saturated fats (safe to cook with because these are stable at high temperatures) including:

Animal fats: lard, dripping, butter, goose fat

Vegetable fats: coconut oil, palm oil, cocoa fat

Unsaturated fats (not safe to cook with as unstable at relatively low temperatures) including:

Fish oils

Vegetable, nut and seed oils e.g. olive, hemp, rape, sunflower, grapeseed, peanut, corn

• Sauerkraut.

Proteins too are zero carb. However, should you eat more than your daily requirement (see Chapter 3 for how to calculate this), the excess will be converted by the liver into sugars and this may knock you out of ketosis.

Appendix 2

Kitchen equipment
– needs over and above the usual

Give us the tools, and we will finish the job.
Sir Winston Leonard Spencer Churchill, 1874 –1965

Keep things simple, quick and easy. The main aim of equipment is to reduce work and washing up. I have as little equipment as I can get away with, so it is all immediately to hand. So, for example my **Nutribullet** lives on the worktop permanently plugged in as I use it daily for PK bread, PK ice cream, soups and smoothies.

Dishwashers wash and rinse plates far more effectively than humans. I recommend **two half-size dishwashers**, one for the dirty loading, one clean for current use. That way you do not waste time or energy unloading and stashing kitchen implements. Crocks and cutlery live permanently in the dishwasher. A canine pre-wash improves the end result since the crusty bits which stick to dishes clearly taste awfully good and prevent clogging up the dishwasher.

I have a **plastic jug** in which kefir resides permanently, albeit alternating between warm kitchen for fermenting and fridge for keeping. That is washed up very occasionally (my record is two months of no washing up).

The **slow cooker** for bone broth (page 177) again is permanently on with occasional washing up – the heat prevents infection. Bones go in and out, cooking vegetable water goes in, so does Sunshine salt and delicious stock results.

I have **Kilner jars** for sauerkraut (page 157) and kvass (page 160).

Appendix 3

Checklist of the PK diet and lifestyle

Have you done all that is needed to put a PK lifestyle in place? Table A3.1 provides a checklist of actions to take (righthand column) with explanations of the problems to be solved.

Table A3.1: Why Western-type diets are so problematic and what we can do about this

Problem	Why this must be addressed	What to do
Addiction to sugar, fruit, caffeine, alcohol, nicotine, cannabis	Addiction masks appetite and we consume for all the wrong reasons. Addictions disturb sleep quality and quantity. Addictions mask symptoms	Depending on the addiction follow the guide below Indulge in your addictions only occasionally and in moderation (See Chapter 20: Feasting and alcohol)
Most Westerners are carbohydrate addicts	Too much carb drives pathology: fatigue, obesity, diabetes, cancer, arteriosclerosis and dementia ('type 3 diabetes')	Get into ketosis – use a ketone breath meter to demonstrate such. In ketosis your muscle and liver glycogen sponges are squeezed dry. That means your body can easily deal with any carbs in the diet. (I am usually in ketosis after breakfast, always in ketosis late afternoon)

Standard Western diets overwhelm the upper gut with carbs	If you overwhelm the ability of the upper gut to digest, then it will ferment and that drives even more pathology: • symptoms include gastritis, reflux, GORD, bloating, burping and foggy brain. • pathology includes inflammation, autoimmunity, toxicity and much more	Do not overeat carbs or proteins. Take vitamin C to bowel tolerance. Fast
	Some carbohydrate is fine – sugars are needed as building blocks (to make DNA, RNA and the energy molecule, ATP) and to detox (glucuronidation), but not too much. The body can make sugar from proteins	Use a ketone breath meter to monitor how you flip in and out of ketosis – that makes sure you are not over-loading with carbs. Get your carbs from vegetables, nuts and seeds. If you never blow positive for ketones, fast until you get a positive test – you need at least one positive test a day
Standard Western diets are low in healthy fats	Fats are highly desirable: • as fuels – the keto-adapted athlete performs 10-15% better. • as building materials for repair and renewal. • for energy delivery to mitochondria. • for the membranes of all cells, especially brain and immune system cells	Eat fatty meats, fish, poultry, duck, eggs, butter. Use lard, dripping, goose fat, coconut oil for cooking. Oils are good for salads and dressings but must not be heated or you create toxic trans fats
Dairy products are meant for young mammals	They are growth promoters – too much of them is a risk for cancer, heart disease, osteoporosis	Cut out all dairy products. The safest dairy products are butter and ghee. Vegan butters, cheeses, coconut milks and coconut yoghurts make superb replacements

Problem	Why this must be addressed	What to do
Western diets are low in fibre	Fibre is needed for: • chewing, which stimulates digestion. • friendly fermentation in the large bowel to produce fuel (short chain fatty acids) and vitamins B and K; this friendly fermentation programmes the immune system and protects against infection. • bulk to allow effortless passage of stools	Eat sufficient fibre until you pass a Bristol Stool Chart number 4, once or twice daily, effortlessly, ideally using a squatty potty. Make the PK linseed bread which is 27% fibre, 2% carb
Western diets are high in processed foods	Processed foods are often addictive (high-carb, low-protein), deficient in micronutrients, toxic with chemicals and low in fibre	Do not eat processed food – eat real foods
Western diets offer little variation	We know that the more diverse the microbes of the gut, the healthier the person overall. Each microbe has a liking for a certain food so a diverse diet supports microbe diversity	Eat as varied a diet as possible; keep ringing the changes. Eat foods that are in season
Addictive Western diets interfere with our being able to tell when we are truly hungry and what foods we need	Our bodies have separate appetites for protein, fat, carbs, salt, micronutrients and possibly more if we can conquer our addictions	Once you have conquered addictions, 'listen' to your appetite for certain foods – if you fancy it you probably need it!
	Pharmacognosy draws us to the foods we need: if we become ill, we develop an appetite for healing herbs, essential oils and other remedies; this is well established in animals and is called zoopharmacognosy	Listen to your appetite, to your brain and to your body; when ill, these appetites may tell you to rest, to fast and to sniff

The standard solution is to adopt a low-calorie diet	Many people half-starve themselves in a misguided attempt to lose weight; this simply makes you tired, cold, foggy-brained and depressed	Make sure you are eating sufficient calories – see Chapter 3 to work out your daily need
Vitamin C deficiency is pandemic	Humans have lost the ability to synthesise vitamin C from sugars so they must consume this essential nutrient, and in much greater quantities if ill	Take vitamin C as ascorbic acid little and often through the day. Everyone's dose is different; take increasing quantities to bowel tolerance or to urine tolerance (test with vitamin C urine test strips). Most people need 5-8 g (5000-8000 mg) daily, much more for acute infections
Micronutrient deficiencies are pandemic	Soils are depleted by modern agriculture and lack of recycling of human compost back to the soils; consequently, foods grown on these soils contain lower levels of all nutrients than formerly	Take a good multivitamin daily and Sunshine salt 5 g
Allergies are common	Irritable bowel syndrome, headaches, asthma and arthritis are often driven by allergy	Cut out common allergens, especially dairy, gluten, yeast Cut out your personal known allergens
Western diets tend to be low in protein	Protein is essential on a daily basis. 'Protein leverage' is when too little protein in the diet stimulates the appetite to eat any food (often high-carb foods) until the protein appetite is satisfied; overeating calories then causes obesity	Calculate your protein requirement as explained in Chapter 3
Snacking: Food being constantly present in the upper gut	This means the stomach never has a chance to heal, repair and restore its normal acidity. Early supper improves sleep quality	Eat all food within a 10-hour window of time: breakfast at 7:30 am, light lunch, supper at 5:30 pm. Do not snack

Problem	Why this must be addressed	What to do
Snacking: Food being constantly present in the mouth	This means the mouth never has a chance to heal, repair and reduce numbers of bacteria. Bacterial overgrowth leads to gum disease and tooth decay	Ditto above. Do not snack
Food being constantly available	Primitive man did not eat three meals a day. Fasting has great benefits: • It switches on autophagy which protects against cancer and degeneration. • It switches on stem cells for new growth and repair. • It clears the foggy brain. • It squeezes dry the glycogen sponge and gets you into ketosis rapidly	Do a 24-hour fast weekly (e.g. skip breakfast and have no lunch for one day a week). Do a 48-hour fast monthly. Perhaps do a longer fast once a year
Western lifestyles are increasingly sedentary	Daily anaerobic exercise will increase muscle bulk; this keeps you strong and increases your basal metabolic rate (BMR). See *Ecological Medicine* Chapter 23: Exercise	Do the right sort of anaerobic exercise – with more muscle you will need to eat more to which I say, 'Jolly good!' I love food and am greedy
Constant dieting/ calorie restriction makes us foggy-brained and miserable	Feasting and alcohol enhance life	Laughter is the best medicine* – have some fun on holidays and special occasions

*'Laughter is the best medicine' is a regular feature in *Reader's Digest* magazine. It consists of medically-based short funny stories or jokes. *Reader's Digest* remains the largest paid-circulation magazine in the world and will be 100 years old on 5 February 2022. Craig used to read this section, and a few others, on his visits to his grandfather. It became a tradition to see Craig sitting in the corner chuckling away at some joke or another. He was allowed to tear out the 'Increase your Word Power' sections and take them home with him.

Appendix 4

Further sources of information

Craig and I are working towards a set of books – the complete library – to give all the Rules of the Game and the Tools of the Trade for our readers to heal themselves with ecological medicine and live to their full potential. So far, we have produced the books listed in Table A4.1.

Table A4.1: The complete library

Ecological Medicine – the antidote to Big Pharma and fast food (this replaces our first book *Sustainable Medicine*)	The 'bible' – an overview of all symptoms, mechanisms and the major Tools of the Trade to prevent and treat all disease from cancer and coronaries to diabetes and dementia
Paleo-Ketogenic – the Why and the How *Prevent and Cure Diabetes – delicious diets not dangerous drugs*	Diet is the starting point to prevent and treat everything
The Infection Game – life is an arms race	Nearly all pathology has an infectious driver. More tools to deal with disease from covid to chronic fatigue
Diagnosis and Treatment of Chronic Fatigue Syndrome and Myalgic Encephalitis – it's mitochondria not hypochondria	A detailed look at energy delivery mechanisms and how to fix them – the pathology of CFS
The Energy Equation – from the naked ape to the knackered ape	Improving energy for the everyday person – a quick and jolly read that is also available as an audiobook

Green Mother – families fit for the future – written with and illustrated by Michelle MoCullagh	The practical application of all the above to pregnancy, birth and child rearing

The complete website

Much of the information in this book and those listed above can be found at www.drmyhill.co.uk. Hits to date (December 2021): total 22,914,260

Facebook pages and other social media

Run by Katie Twinn and Craig Robinson for people with CFS and ME:
> Support for followers of Dr Myhill's protocol:
> www.facebook.com/groups/435645003161721

> See here for all my social media platforms:
> https://drmyhill.co.uk/wiki/My_Social_Media_Presence

Online workshops

At these, any person can listen to and cross-examine Dr Myhill directly on any aspect of medicine. This is especially popular with CFS/ME patients:
> https://drmyhill.co.uk/wiki/Workshops_for_Ecological_Medicine

Other websites

Natural Health Worldwide
https://naturalhealthworldwide.com
Here you can find like-minded doctors and therapists, and access medical tests directly.

The British Society for Ecological Medicine (BSEM)
www.bsem.org.uk
Here practitioners can meet like-minded doctors and therapists. Dr Myhill is a

long-standing committee member, helps with doctor training and runs mentoring groups for interested doctors.

The Association of Naturopathic Practitioners
https://theanp.co.uk/
This is a useful way to find a practitioner. Dr Myhill often does webinars for members.

The College of Naturopathic Medicine
www.naturopathy-uk.com
CNM offers courses through which you can learn about naturopathic and ecological medicine and study to become a practitioner. Dr Myhill helps with some of the training courses and has recently been appointed a Patron.

Glossary

Adrenal gland problems

The adrenal gland is the 'gear box' of our car responsible for matching energy demand with energy delivery. It is additionally responsible for controlling the amount of inflammation in the body. It achieves this by secreting adrenaline (the short-term response, measured in seconds and minutes), followed by cortisol (a medium-term response measured in minutes and hours), followed by DHEA (dehydroepiandrosterone – a longer-term stress hormone).

The Hungarian physiologist Hans Selye showed that if you stressed rats, their adrenal glands enlarged to produce more stress hormones (including cortisol and DHEA) to allow the rat to cope with that stress. If the rat had a break and a rest, then the adrenal gland would return to its normal size and recover. However, if the rat was stressed without a break or a rest, he would be apparently all right for some time, but then suddenly collapse and die. When Selye looked at the adrenal glands at this point, they were shrivelled up. The glands had become exhausted.

The current Western way of life is for people to push themselves more and more. Many can cope with a great deal of stress, but everybody has their breaking point. The adrenal gland is responsible for the body's hormonal response to this stress. It produces adrenaline, which stimulates the instant stress hormone response ('fight or flight' reaction), and cortisol and DHEA, which create the short- and long-term stress hormone responses respectively. When the gland becomes exhausted, chronic fatigue develops and tests of adrenal function typically show low levels of cortisol and DHEA. DHEA has only recently been studied because it had not been realised that it had any important actions.

All steroid hormone synthesis starts with cholesterol The first biochemical step takes place in mitochondria where there is a conversion to pregnenolone. The body can then shunt from pregnenolone either into a stress or catabolic mode (to cortisol) or a rebuilding mode (anabolic hormones such as DHEA, testosterone and oestrogen).

Adrenaline (epinephrine)

Adrenaline is the instant stress response hormone that drives our fight or flight reaction. This reaction is characterised by intense arousal (sometimes to the point of anxiety or panic), with a faster heart rate, high blood pressure, higher blood sugar level and sometimes even minor tremor. This is the stress hormone which allows us to move up a gear, sometimes perhaps into overdrive, even in order to kill, within a stressful situation. An obvious evolutionary cause of such stress would be to be hunted by a predator. In our modern, safer lives, I suspect that the commonest stress is falling blood sugar levels and this release of adrenaline is a central part of metabolic syndrome.

Allergy

Allergy is the great mimic. In some ways the immune system is not very clever. It can react to things in only one way – that is, with inflammation. Inflammation causes redness, swelling, pain, heat and loss of function. When you look at a diseased area, you can see those signs, but it does not tell you what the cause is. So, for example, looking at an area of inflamed skin you may not be able to tell if it has been infected, sun-burnt or frozen, had acid spilled on it, or is responding allergically, or whatever. Again, seeing a person with hay fever you may not be able to distinguish this from a head cold. Hay fever sufferers may get a fever too.

You can be allergic to anything under the sun, including the sun. For practical purposes, allergies are split up into allergies to foods, chemicals (including drugs) and inhalants (pollens and micro-organisms such as bacteria, mites, etc).

People with undiagnosed food allergy often initially present with symptoms due to inflammation in the gut (irritable bowel syndrome) and inflammation in the brain (mood swings, depression or brain fog in adults, or hyperactivity in children). However, the inflammation can occur anywhere in the body, resulting in asthma, rhinitis, eczema, arthritis and muscle pain, cystitis or vaginitis, or a combination of symptoms.

Antioxidants

What allows us to live and our bodies to function are billions of chemical reactions in the body which occur every second. These are essential to produce energy, which drives all the processes of life such as nervous function, movement, heart function, digestion and so on. If all these enzyme reactions invariably occurred perfectly, there would be no need for an antioxidant system.

However, even our own enzyme systems make mistakes and the process of producing energy in mitochondria is highly active. When mistakes occur, free radicals are produced. Essentially, a free radical is a molecule with an unpaired electron; it is highly reactive and to stabilise its own structure, it will literally stick on to anything. That 'anything' could be a cell membrane, a protein, a fat, a piece of DNA, or whatever. In sticking on to something, it denatures that something so that it has to be replaced. This means having free radicals is extremely damaging to the body and therefore the body has evolved a system to mop up these free radicals before they have a chance to do such damage, and this is called our antioxidant system. There are many substances in the body which act as antioxidants, but the three most important **frontline antioxidants** are:

- **co-enzyme Q10.** This is the most important antioxidant inside mitochondria and also a vital molecule in oxidative phosphorylation. Co-Q10 deficiency may also cause oxidative phosphorylation to go slow because it is the most important receiver and donor of electrons in oxidative phosphorylation. People with low levels of Co-Q10 have low levels of energy.
- **superoxide dismutase (SODase).** This is the most important super oxide scavenger in muscles (zinc and copper SODase inside cells; manganese SODase inside mitochondria; and zinc and copper SODase outside cells).
- **glutathione peroxidase**. This enzyme is dependent on selenium and glutathione, a 3-amino acid polypeptide, and a vital free-radical scavenger in the bloodstream.

These molecules are present in parts of a million and are in the frontline process of absorbing free radicals. They give up their own electrons and, in the process, they neutralise the unpaired electrons in free radicals. This process continues, via complex sets of reactions, along a chain of antioxidants, such as vitamins A and E, before the ultimate electron donor, vitamin C, gives up its electrons in the same way.

Autoimmunity

Autoimmunity occurs when the immune system has made a mistake. The immune system has a difficult job to do, because it has to distinguish between molecules which are dangerous to the body and molecules which are safe. Sometimes it gets its wires crossed and starts making antibodies against molecules which are 'safe'. For some people this results in allergies, which is a useless inflammation against 'safe' foreign molecules. For others this results in autoimmunity, which is a useless inflammation against the body's own molecules. These are acquired problems – we know that because they become much more common with age. It is likely we are seeing more autoimmunity because of Western lifestyles, diets and pollution. Chemicals, especially heavy metals, get stuck onto cells and change their 'appearance' to the immune system and thereby switch on inappropriate reactions.

Brain fog/Foggy brain

What I mean by brain fog is:
- Poor short-term memory.
- Difficulty learning new things.
- Poor mental stamina and concentration – there may be difficulty reading a book or following a film story or following a line of argument.
- Difficulty finding the right word.
- Thinking one word but saying another.

What allows the brain to work quickly and efficiently is its energy supply. If this is impaired in any way, then the brain will go slow. Initially, the symptoms would be of foggy brain, but if symptoms progress, we end up with dementia. We all see this in our everyday life, with the effect of alcohol being the best example. Short-term exposure

214

gives us a deliciously foggy brain – we stop caring, we stop worrying, it alleviates anxiety. However, it also removes our drive to do things, our ability to remember; it impairs judgement and our ability to think clearly. Medium-term exposure results in mood swings and anxiety (only alleviated by more alcohol). Longer-term use could result in severe depression and then dementia – examples include Korsakoff's psychosis and Wernike's encephalopathy.

Carbohydrate

All vegetable material (grains, pulses, vegetables, salads, fruit, berries, nuts and seeds) contain carbohydrates. These are comprised of:

- Simple monosaccharides and disaccharides. (They all taste sweet, and we call them sugars.)
- Polysaccharides. (These are starches, such as from grain flours or potato.)
- Complex polysaccharides (which we call vegetable fibre).

The sugars and starches are easily digested in our gut and are readily absorbed.

Vegetable fibre cannot be digested by human enzymes; it must be fermented by friendly bacteria in the large bowel. It is fermented to form short chain fatty acids, which are a useful fuel for the body, and they do not affect blood sugar levels. This is what makes high-fibre vegetables such desirable foods.

When looking at food labels, take care. When we 'count carbs', we are looking for the Net Carbohydrate figure – that is Total Carbohydrate MINUS Fibre. When reading food labels, one must understand the difference between how things are disclosed in the US and the EU and UK. For example, if an item, in America, contains 5 grams of Total Carbohydrates, out of which 2 grams consist of Dietary Fibre, then the Net Carbohydrate content of this product is 3 grams (5 grams minus 2 grams). In the UK 'Net Carbohydrates' are already calculated within nutritional labels. Sugars and Starches are disclosed as one entity ('Carbohydrate') and dietary fibre is separately labelled as 'Fibre'. Hence there is no need to calculate Net Carbohydrate content for a product that follows EU labelling rules. For example, if an item from an EU country is said to contain 3 grams of Carbohydrate and 2 grams of Fibre, then the amount of carbohydrates that will affect blood sugar levels is 3 grams. But do always check and be sure!

Chemical poisoning

The diagnosis of chemical poisoning is suspected from a history of exposures resulting in typical clinical syndromes and confirmed by the appropriate medical tests. There is a series of criteria to be fulfilled to make a confident clinical diagnosis of poisoning by chemicals. The criteria are:

1. The subject was fit and well prior to chemical exposures.
2. There is evidence of exposure to the putative chemicals and toxins.
3. The subject initially developed local symptoms which became worse with repeated exposures.
4. With repeated exposures a typical clinical picture emerges characterised by chronic fatigue syndrome, immune disruption (allergies, autoimmunity, susceptibility to infections), accelerated ageing (so the sufferer gets diseases before their time), neurodegeneration, diabetes and cancer.
5. Similar patterns of disease are seen in other people working under similar conditions.
6. There is similar factual evidence from other individuals who have been poisoned, such as the Gulf War veterans, sheep-dip-poisoned farmers and aerotoxic pilots.
7. There is laboratory evidence of poisoning and effects of that poisoning.
8. There are no other possible explanations for this pattern of symptoms.
9. There is a response to treatment with clinical improvements as a result of detoxification and nutritional and immune support.

Co-enzyme Q10

See antioxidants.

Cortisol

Cortisol is a hormone released by the adrenal gland in response to stress. Essentially, adrenaline is the immediate response, cortisol the medium-term response and DHEA the long-term response. Between these three hormones the body can gear up to stress, maintain that stress response for the required duration, and then normality is restored as the levels of these hormones drop back to normal.

Detoxification

As part of normal metabolism, the body produces toxins which have to be eliminated, otherwise they poison the system. Therefore, the body has evolved a mechanism for getting rid of these toxins and the methods that it uses are as follows:

- Antioxidant system – for mopping up free radicals. See Antioxidants.
- The liver – detoxification by oxidation and conjugation (amino acids, sulphur compounds, glucuronide, glutathione, etc) for excretion in urine.
- Fat-soluble toxins can be excreted in the bile. The problem here is that many of these are recycled because they are reabsorbed in the gut.
- Sweating – many toxins and heavy metals can be lost through the skin.
- Dumping chemicals in hair, nails and skin, which are then shed.

This system has worked perfectly well for thousands of years. Problems now arise because of toxins which we are absorbing from the outside world. This is inevitable since we live in equilibrium with the outside world. The problem is that these toxins (such as alcohol) may overwhelm the system for detoxification, or they may be impossible to break down (e.g. silicone and organochlorines), or they may get stuck in fatty organs and cell membranes and so not be accessible to the liver for detoxification (for example, many volatile organic compounds). We all carry these toxins as a result of living in our polluted world.

We can help our bodies detoxify by:

- eating a PK diet - increasing the fibre content of food and the bacterial numbers in the gut also facilitates detoxification
- taking a basic package of nutritional supplements – see Chapter 2
- heating regimes
- improving antioxidant status
- see https://drmyhill.co.uk/wiki/Detoxification_-_an_overview

Fermenting gut – 'upper fermenting gut'

The human gut is almost unique amongst mammals: the upper gut is a near-sterile, digesting, carnivorous gut (like a dog's or a cat's) to deal with meat and fat, whilst the lower gut (large bowel or colon) is full of bacteria and is a fermenting, vegetarian gut (like a horse's or cow's) to digest vegetables and fibre. From an evolutionary perspective this has been a highly successful strategy – it allows Inuits to live on fat and protein and other people to survive on pure vegan diets. Problems arose when humans learned to cook and to farm. This allowed them to access new foods – namely, pulses, grains and root vegetables. These need cooking to be digestible. From an evolutionary perspective this has been highly successful and allowed the population of humans to increase at a great rate. However, carbohydrates have the potential to be fermented in the upper gut with problems arising as detailed below.

The stomach, duodenum and small intestine should be almost free from micro-organisms (bacteria, yeasts and parasites – that is, 'microbes'). This is achieved by eating a PK diet, having an acidic stomach which digests protein efficiently and kills the acid-sensitive microbes; then an alkaline duodenum, which kills the alkali-sensitive microbes with bicarbonate; then bile salts (which are also toxic to microbes) and pancreatic enzymes to further digest protein, fats and carbohydrates. The small intestine does more digesting and also absorbs the amino acids, fatty acids, glycerol and simple sugars that result.

Anaerobic bacteria (bacteria that do not use oxygen), largely bacteroides, flourish in the large bowel, where foods that cannot be digested upstream are then fermented to produce many substances that are highly beneficial to the body. Bacteroides ferment soluble fibre to produce short-chain fatty acids – over 500 kcal of energy a day can be generated. This also creates heat to help keep us warm. The human body is made up of 10 trillion cells, yet in our gut we have 100 trillion microbes or more – that is, 10 times as many. Bacteria make up 60% of dry stool weight. There are over 500 different species, but 99% of microbes are from 30–40 species.

In people not eating a PK diet, there are bacteria, yeasts and possibly other parasites existing in the upper gut (stomach, duodenum and small intestine), which means that foods are fermented there instead of being digested. When foods get fermented this can cause symptoms and problems for many reasons such as:
- wind, bloating, heartburn and other digestive problems (so-called irritable bowel syndrome)
- malabsorption
- production of toxins through fermentation or enhanced absorption of toxic metals
- allergy to microbes in the gut (inflammatory bowel disease)
- allergy to microbes at distant sites in the body, manifesting as arthritis, interstitial

cystitis, asthma, urticaria, PMR and many others
- in the longer term – cancer, diverticulitis.

Glycogen sponge

All the products resulting from food being digested and then absorbed in the gut pass via the portal vein to the liver. These products are toxic. So, for example, if this toxic load were to pass straight into the systemic bloodstream, we would rapidly lose consciousness and succumb. This occurs in liver failure. One of the toxins in the portal vein is sugar. This is like the petrol in our car – essential for it to run but highly dangerous in large amounts. The liver glycogen sponge prevents the tsunami of sugar in the portal vein from getting into the systemic bloodstream by way of a mopping-up operation. The liver achieves this by rapidly shunting sugar in the blood into the more complex storage form, glycogen, and holding it safely in store, from where it can be used as a pantry when blood sugar levels fall. In this respect the liver has a sponge-like effect. Should sugar levels in the systemic bloodstream fall, then the glycogen sponge can correct this by 'squeezing dry'.

Glycogen can also be stored in the muscles so these too can act as glycogen sponges to be squeezed dry, as needed.

Gulf War syndrome (GWS)

GWS is the archetypal environmental illness suffered by any person involved in the Gulf Wars. It was caused by a combination of factors, including:
- Immune insult caused by many different vaccinations (up to 14 in some soldiers) given on the same day.
- Chemical warfare – organophosphate chemical weapons were used in the Gulf, notably sarin.
- Biological warfare – infectious agents were sprayed onto the troops; the organism was *Mycoplasma incognito*.
- Pyridostigmine – this is the 'antidote' to organophosphate poisoning but is toxic in its own right.
- Organophosphate pesticides, used for control of sand flies and other insects, were

weekly sprayed onto tents and all uniforms were dipped in them.

- Fumes from oil-well fires.
- Depleted uranium resulting in radioactive exposures.
- Water from drinking and showering was often stored in tanks usually used for oil and diesel.

This was the most environmentally polluting war in history. Veterans tell me that the chemical alarms were constantly going off, but the usual response was to switch the alarm off! Many of the soldiers who came back from the Gulf War with GWS are suffering, amongst other things, from a chronic infection caused by *Mycoplasma incognito*. This was developed as part of germ warfare, and it may be that many thousands of the veterans are infected. Treatment is with high dose doxycycline (200 milligrams daily for six weeks, with further cycles given subsequently). To find out more about mycoplasmal infections and how to test for them, visit the website of the Institute of Molecular Medicine (www.immed.org/).

Hypoglycaemia (see also the mis-named 'Ketogenic hypoglycaemia')

'Hypoglycaemia' is the term used for blood sugar being at too low a level. To explain how this happens it is necessary to describe how sugar levels are controlled.

It is critically important for the body to maintain blood sugar levels within a narrow range. If the blood sugar level falls too low, energy supply to all tissues, particularly the brain, is impaired. However, if blood sugar levels rise too high, then this is very damaging to arteries and the long-term effect of arterial disease is heart disease and strokes. This is caused by sugar sticking to proteins and fats to make AGEs (advanced glycation end-products) which accelerate the ageing process.

Normally, the liver controls blood sugar levels. It can convert glycogen stores inside the liver to release sugar into the bloodstream minute by minute in a carefully regulated way to cope with body demands, which may fluctuate from minute to minute. Excess sugar flooding into the system after a meal can be mopped up by muscles, but only so long as there is space there to act as a sponge. This occurs when we exercise. This system of control works perfectly well until we upset it by eating a high-carb diet and/or not exercising. Eating excessive sugar at one meal, or excessive refined carbohydrate, which is rapidly digested into sugar, can suddenly overwhelm the muscle and the liver's normal control of blood sugar levels.

We evolved over millions of years eating a diet that was very low in sugar and had no refined carbohydrate. Control of blood sugar therefore largely occurred as a result of eating this PK diet and exercising vigorously in the course of daily life, so any excessive sugar in the blood was quickly burned off. Nowadays the situation is different: we eat large amounts of sugar and refined carbohydrate and do not exercise sufficiently to burn off this excess sugar. The body therefore has to cope with this excessive sugar load by other mechanisms.

When food is digested, the sugars and other digestive products go straight from the gut in the portal vein to the liver, where they should all be mopped up by the liver and processed accordingly. If excessive sugar or refined carbohydrate overwhelms the liver, the sugar spills over into the systemic circulation. If not absorbed by muscle glycogen stores, high blood sugar results, which is extremely damaging to arteries. If we were exercising hard, this would be quickly burned off. However, if we are not, then other mechanisms of control are brought into play. The key player here is insulin, a hormone secreted by the pancreas. This is very good at bringing blood sugar levels down and it does so by shunting the sugar into fat. Indeed, this includes the 'bad' cholesterol LDL. There is then a rebound effect and blood sugars may well go too low – in other words, hypoglycaemia occurs. Low blood sugar is also dangerous to the body because the energy supplied to all tissues is impaired.

Subconsciously, people quickly work out that eating more sugar alleviates these symptoms, but of course they invariably overdo things; the blood sugar level then goes high, and they end up on a roller-coaster ride of their blood sugar level going up and down throughout the day. Ultimately, this leads to 'metabolic syndrome' or 'syndrome X' – a major cause of disability and death in Western societies, since it is the forerunner of diabetes, obesity, cardiovascular disease, degenerative conditions and cancer.

Hypothyroidism – underactive thyroid

An underactive thyroid is a very common cause of fatigue, often as a knock-on effect of a general suppression of the hypothalamic-pituitary-adrenal axis – that is, the coordinated functioning of those three glands. Symptoms of hypothyroidism arise for four reasons –

either the gland itself fails (primary thyroid failure), or the pituitary gland which drives the thyroid gland into action under-functions, or there is failure to convert inactive thyroxine (T4) to its active form (T3), or there is thyroid-hormone receptor resistance. The symptoms of these four problems are the same, but blood tests show different patterns:

- In **primary thyroid failure**, blood tests show high levels of thyroid stimulating hormone (TSH) and low levels of T4 and T3.
- In **pituitary failure**, blood tests show low levels of TSH, T4 and T3.
- If there is a **conversion problem**, TSH and T4 may be normal, but T3 is low.
- In **thyroid hormone receptor resistance**, there is a high TSH, high T4 and high T3.

There is another problem too, which is that the so-called 'normal range' of T4 is probably set too low. I know this because many patients with low normal T4 often improve substantially when they are started on thyroid supplements to bring levels up to the top end of the normal range.

Inflammation

Inflammation is an essential part of our survival package. From an evolutionary perspective, the biggest killer of Homo sapiens (apart from Homo sapiens) has been infection, with cholera claiming a third of all deaths, ever. The body has to be alert to the possibility of any infection, to all of which it responds with inflammation. However, inflammation is metabolically expensive and inherently destructive. It has to be, in order to kill infections by bacteria, viruses, parasites or whatever. For example, part of the immune defence involves a 'scorched earth' policy – tissue immediately around an area of infection is destroyed so there is nothing for the invader to parasitise.

The mechanism by which the immune system kills these infections is by firing free radicals at them. However, if it fires too many free radicals, then this 'friendly fire' will damage the body itself. Therefore, for inflammation to be effective it must be switched on, targeted, localised and then switched off. This entails extremely complex immune responses; clearly, there is great potential for things to go wrong.

Inflammation is also involved in the healing process. Where there is damage by trauma, there will be dead cells. Inflammation is necessary to clear away these dead cells and lay down new tissues.

Inflammation is characterised by heat and redness (heat alone is antiseptic), combined with swelling, pain and loss of function, which immobilises the area being attacked by the immune system. This is necessary because physical movement will tend to massage the infection to other sites.

If one looks at life from the point of view of the immune system, it has a very difficult balancing act to manage. Too little reaction and we die from infection; too much reaction is metabolically expensive and damaging. If switched on inappropriately, the immune system has the power to kill us within seconds, an example of this being anaphylaxis.

Ketosis

Ketosis is a metabolic state where the majority of the body's energy supply is derived from ketone bodies in the blood. This is in contrast with a state of glycolysis where blood glucose provides the majority of the energy supply.

Ketoacidosis

Diabetic ketoacidosis is a potentially life-threatening complication caused by a lack of insulin in the body. This may occur if the body is unable to use blood sugar (glucose) as a source of fuel. Instead, the body breaks down fat as an alternative source of fuel and because of the severity of the situation in diabetic ketoacidosis, this can lead to a dangerously high build-up of ketones.

Ketosis, the breaking down of fat, is desirable and an entirely different thing.

Keto-adaptation

Keto-adaptation is being able to switch from burning sugar and carbs as a source of fuel to burning fat and fibre, giving the individual much longer-lasting energy and greater stamina.

Ketogenic hypoglycaemia – also known as 'keto flu'

This is described in detail in Chapter 5.

Leaky gut

Leaky gut means that substances which should be held in the gut leak out through the gut wall. This causes many problems:

- Hydrogen ions (i.e. acid) cannot be concentrated in the stomach, leading to hypochlorhydria – a lack of stomach acid. This causes malabsorption of minerals and vitamin B12. Hypochlorhydria is a major risk factor for fermenting gut since acid helps to sterilise the upper gut. It also is an essential part of protein digestion.
- Allergy - Normally one expects foods to be completely broken down into amino acids (from protein), essential fatty acids and glycerol (from fats) and single sugars, or 'monosaccharides' (from carbohydrates). The undigested foods stay in the gut and the small, digested molecules pass through the gut wall into the portal bloodstream and on to the liver where they are dealt with. However, leaky gut means food particles get absorbed before they have been properly digested. This means large food molecules get into the bloodstream. These large molecules are 'interesting' to the immune system, which may mistake them for viruses and/or bacteria. In this event, it may attack these harmless molecules, either with antibodies or directly with immune cells. This causes inflammation. Inflammation in the gut causes diseases of the gut. Inflammation elsewhere can cause almost any symptom you care to mention. It may switch on allergy and/or auto-immunity – that is, it is potentially a disease-amplifying process.
- Another problem with small, digested molecules or polypeptides getting into the bloodstream is that these molecules may be biologically active. Some of them act as hormone mimics, which can affect levels of glucose in the blood or blood pressure. This is akin to throwing a handful of sand into a finely tuned machine – it makes a real mess of homeostatic (balancing) mechanisms of controlling body activities.

Magnesium

Magnesium is an essential mineral required for at least 300 different enzyme systems in the body. It is centrally involved in the energy delivery systems of the body – that is, the mitochondria.

Red blood cell levels of magnesium are almost invariably low in my ME patients and very many benefit from magnesium by injection.

I believe that a low red-cell magnesium is a symptom of mitochondrial failure. It is the job of mitochondria to produce ATP for cell metabolism, and about 40% of all mitochondrial output goes into maintaining calcium/magnesium and sodium/potassium ion pumps. I suspect that when mitochondria fail, these pumps malfunction and therefore calcium leaks into cells and magnesium leaks out. This, of course, compounds the underlying mitochondrial failure because calcium is toxic to mitochondria and magnesium necessary for normal mitochondrial function. This is just one of the many vicious cycles we see in patients with fatigue syndromes. The reason for giving magnesium by injection is in order to reduce the work of the calcium/magnesium ion pump by reducing the concentration gradient across cell membranes.

Malabsorption

The job of the gut is to absorb the goodness from food. To do this, it first has to reduce food particles to a size which allows the digestive enzymes to get at them; then it has to provide the correct acidity then alkalinity for enzymes to work, produce the necessary enzymes and emulsifying agent (bile salts), and move the food along the gut. Lastly, the large bowel allows growth of bacteria for a final digestive/fermentative process and water extraction.

The gut has a particularly difficult job because it has to identify foods that are safe from potentially dangerous microbes (most are not dangerous but positively beneficial). This explains why 90% of the immune system is associated with the gut. The inoculation of the gut with these gut-friendly microbes takes place in the first few minutes following birth.

Anything which goes wrong with any of these processes can cause malabsorption. Malabsorption means that the body does not get the raw materials for normal everyday work and repair. Consequently, there is the potential for much more to go wrong.

Metabolic inflexibility

Metabolic inflexibility is the condition that arises when the body cannot switch from burning sugars and starches as its fuel source to running on fibres and fats. This is the opposite of keto-adaptation – that is, the metabolic condition which arises when the body is powering itself from fat and ketones. This inflexibility can give rise to ketogenic hypoglycaemia – see above and Chapter 5.

Metabolic syndrome

This is the clinical picture which arises when the body powers itself predominantly with sugars and carbohydrates. There is a loss of control over blood sugar levels. The conventional definition of metabolic syndrome only occurs in an advanced state of such – that is, when there is a combination of abdominal (central) obesity (i.e. being apple shaped), high blood pressure, high fasting sugar, high triglycerides and low levels of friendly high-density lipoprotein (HDL). My advice is not to wait for these nasty and damaging features to emerge, but to tackle the metabolic syndrome early by eating a PK diet as described in this book.

Minerals

You could argue that we all die ultimately from mineral and vitamin deficiencies. People who traditionally live to a great age are often found living in areas watered by streams from glaciers. Glaciers are lakes of ice which have spent the previous few thousand years crunching up rocks. Therefore, the waters coming from the glaciers are rich in minerals. This is used not just to drink but to irrigate crops and to bathe in. These people therefore have had excellent levels of micronutrients throughout life. Given the right raw materials, things do not go wrong in the body and ageing is slowed. For example:

- Low magnesium and selenium are a risk factor for heart disease
- Low selenium increases the risk of cancer
- Copper is necessary to make elastic tissue – deficiency causes weaknesses in arteries, leading to aneurysms
- Low chromium increases the risk of diabetes
- Good antioxidant status (vitamins A, C, E and selenium) slows the ageing process
- The superoxide dismutase enzymes (which counteract oxygen free radicals) require zinc, copper and manganese to function
- Iodine is necessary to make thyroid hormones and is highly protective against breast disease

- The immune system needs a huge range of minerals to work well, especially zinc, selenium and magnesium
- Boron is highly protective against arthritis
- Magnesium is required in at least 300 enzyme systems
- Zinc is needed for normal brain development – a deficiency at a critical stage of development causes dyslexia
- Any deficiency of selenium, zinc, copper or magnesium can cause infertility
- Iron prevents anaemia
- Molybdenum is necessary to detox sulphites.

The secret of success is to copy Nature. Sunshine salt (page 147) provides all these minerals in the correct physiological doses. Civilisation and Western diets have brought great advantages, but at the same time are responsible for escalating death rates from cancer, heart disease and dementia. I want the best of both worlds. I like my warm kitchen, fridge, wood-burning cooker, computer and telly, but I want to eat and live in the environment in which primitive man thrived.

Nickel (Ni)

Nickel is a nasty, toxic metal and a known carcinogen. It is one of the metals we see most commonly in toxicity tests – it appears stuck onto DNA, stuck on to translocator protein and is often present in blood at high levels. Nickel is a problem because biochemically it 'looks' like zinc. Zinc deficiency is very common in people eating Western diets, and so if the body needs zinc and it is not there, it will use look-alike nickel instead. But nickel does not do the job and, indeed, gets in the way of normal biochemistry. Zinc is an essential co-factor in many enzyme systems, from alcohol dehydrogenase to zinc carboxypeptidase, and so there is enormous potential for harm from nickel.

Nickel sensitivity is very common and often diagnosed from rashes from jewellery, zips, watches etc. What we know from people with chemical sensitivity is that they often have toxic loads of those things they are sensitive to. So, nickel sensitivity often equates with nickel toxicity.

Nickel is unavoidable if you live a Western lifestyle. Many industrial and other processes release nickel into the atmosphere:

- Stainless steel contains 14% nickel; this includes cookware and eating utensils. Use cast iron pans, glass or ceramic
- Jewellery used because it is such a versatile, malleable metal. It is well-absorbed with piercing
- Catalytic converters in cars release fine particulate nickel into the atmosphere – so fine that it cannot be filtered out by the lining of the bronchus, so it is well-absorbed by inhalation and easily gets into blood vessels. Here it triggers inflammation and arterial disease
- Cigarette smoke
- Medical prostheses such as artificial hip joints.

Organophosphate (OP) poisoning

OP poisoning is a remarkably common but under-diagnosed problem because we are all constantly exposed to organophosphates, including glyphosate – this (Round-up is the best-known product) is generally regarded as safe, but this is not so.

Different people have different symptoms of OP poisoning and these symptoms depend partly on how much OP they have been exposed to, whether they have had single massive exposure or chronic sub-lethal exposure, whether it has been combined with other chemicals, and how good their body is at coping with toxic chemicals. Symptoms divide into the following categories:

- **No obvious symptoms at all** – A government-sponsored study at the Institute of Occupational Medicine, UK, that looked at farmers who regularly handled OPs but who were complaining of no symptoms, showed that they suffered from mild brain damage. Their ability to think clearly and problem solve was impaired.
- **Sheep dip 'flu (mild acute poisoning** – This is a 'flu-like illness which follows exposure to OPs. Sometimes the farmer just has a bit of a headache, feels unusually tired or finds s/he can't think clearly. This may just last a few hours to a few days and the sufferer recovers completely. Most sufferers do not realise that they have been poisoned and put any symptoms down to a hard day's work. It can occur after dipping, but some farmers will get symptoms after the slightest exposure, such as visiting markets and inhaling OP fumes from fleeces.
- **Acute organophosphate poisoning** – This is the syndrome recognised by doctors

and Poisons Units. Symptoms occur within 24 hours of exposure and include collapse, breathing problems, sweating, diarrhoea, vomiting, excessive salivation, heart dysrhythmias, extreme anxiety etc. Treatment is with atropine. You have to have a large dose of OP to have this effect (such as, drink some of the dip!) and so this syndrome is rarely seen.

- **Intermediate syndrome** – This occurs one to three weeks after exposure and is characterised by weakness of shoulder, neck and upper leg muscles. It is rarely diagnosed because it goes unrecognised.
- **Long-term chronic effects** – These symptoms develop in some susceptible individuals. They can either occur following a single massive exposure, or after several years of regular sub-lethal exposure to OPs. Essentially there is an acceleration of the normal ageing process, with arterial disease, heart disease, cancer and dementia presenting at a young age.

Osteoporosis

Osteoporosis is a modern disease of Western society. Primitive societies eating PK diets do not suffer from osteoporosis. So, the underlying principle for avoiding osteoporosis is that we should mimic primitive cultures eating a PK diet and living as toxin-free a life as possible. This does not mean you need to run around half naked in a rabbit-skin loin cloth depriving yourself of the pleasures of 21st century Western life. We need to cherry-pick from the good things of all civilisations.

To make good quality bone you need the raw materials (PK diet and supplements), the ability to absorb minerals (an acid stomach) and the drive to lay these down in bone (exercise, vitamin D). I have collected before and after bone density scans of 14 patients doing these regimes. In all cases, the bone density has remained the same or increased. So, whilst the numbers are small the statistics are powerful.

Dairy products and calcium supplements alone make osteoporosis worse. This is because calcium in isolation blocks the absorption of other essential minerals, such as magnesium. Vitamin D is the key to calcium – it promotes the absorption of calcium (and magnesium) and ensures its deposition in bone.

The medical profession would have us believe that the only important constituent of bone is calcium. Actually, bone is made up of many different minerals, including magnesium, calcium, potassium, boron, silicon, manganese, iron, zinc, copper, chromium, strontium and maybe others. For its formation it also requires a whole range of vitamins, essential fatty acids and amino acids.

Pain

Although pain seems like 'a pain', actually it is essential for our survival. Pain protects us from ourselves. It prevents us from damaging our bodies. Indeed, people who are born with no pain perception look as if they have been traumatised – they are covered in cuts, bruises and sores, because they are unaware that they are damaging themselves. Pain is the local method of avoiding damage – it makes us protect the affected part of the body and keep it still so that healing and repair can take place. If pain becomes more general-ised, then it is accompanied by fatigue. What this means is that chronic pain and chronic fatigue go hand in hand and therefore so should treatment. We learn through experience what is painful; this makes us avoid those painful experiences and therefore protects our bodies.

Although it is desirable to learn about pain, this can also cause problems because if the underlying causes of the pain are not identified we 'learn' more pain. In the ideal situation, we damage our bodies with say a cut or bruise and the local pain makes us care for that damaged area by protecting it and keeping it still so that healing and repair can take place. With healing the pain goes. If the root source of the pain is not identified, it creates a problem because then the pain increases. The body naturally thinks that increasing pain means we will take more care, identify the source of the pain, keep the limb more still and therefore the body winds up the pain signal to try to elicit the appro-priate response. Effectively we learn to feel more pain because there is an upgrading of this pain response. This is not a psychological effect – this actually occurs within the cells themselves. This makes it very important to identify causes of pain early on in any disease process and allow time for healing and repair, otherwise the pain will get worse.

Pancreatic function

The pancreas is a large gland which lies behind the stomach and upper gut. It has two major functions of clinical importance. Firstly, it acts as an endocrine organ to produce insulin and other hormones essential for the control of blood sugar. Secondly, it has an exocrine function to produce enzymes essential for the digestion of food. These enzymes include those to digest proteins, fats and starches, and to work best they need an alkali environment as is found in the small intestine courtesy of the pancreas. When food is present in the duodenum and jejunum (the first two sections of the small intestine), the gall bladder contracts, sending in a bolus of bile salts which combine with bicarbonate and pancreatic enzymes to allow digestion to take place.

If the pancreas does not produce sufficient digestive enzymes and bicarbonate, then foods will not be digested. This can lead to problems downstream. Firstly, foods may be fermented instead of being digested and this can produce the symptom of bloating due to wind, together with metabolites such as various alcohols, hydrogen sulphide and other toxic compounds. Secondly, foods are not fully broken down so they cannot be absorbed, and this can result in malabsorption.

Where there is severe pancreatic dysfunction, it is obvious because the stools themselves become greasy and fatty, foul smelling, bulky and difficult to flush away. Where there is malabsorption of fat, there will be malabsorption of essential fatty acids such as the omega-3 and omega-6 fatty acids, and there will be malabsorption of fat-soluble vitamins such as vitamins A, D, E and K.

If foods are poorly digested, this results in large antigenically interesting molecules appearing downstream, which alerts the immune system and could switch on allergies – that is, poor digestion of food is a risk factor for allergy.

Where there is poor pancreatic function digestive aids can be very helpful. I use pancreatic enzymes together with magnesium carbonate 90 minutes after food (not with food since we need a 90-minute window of time of acidity for stomach function). High-dose pancreatic enzymes have revolutionised the treatment of cystic fibrosis.

Probiotics

In a normal situation, free from antiseptics, antibiotics, high-carbohydrate diets, bottle feeding, hormones and other such accoutrements of modern western life, the gut microbiome is safe. Babies start life in their mother's womb with a sterile gut (although interestingly there is some evidence that their gut becomes inoculated before birth through transfer of microbes across the placenta). During the process of birth, they become inoculated with bacteria from the birth canal and perineum. These bacteria are largely bacteroides which cannot survive for more than a few minutes outside the human gut. This inoculation is enhanced through breast-feeding because the first milk, namely colostrum, is a highly desirable substrate for these bacteria to flourish. We now know that this is an essential part of immune programming. Indeed, 90% of the immune system is gut associated.

These essential probiotics programme the immune system so that they accept them and learn what is beneficial. A healthy gut microbiome therefore is highly protective against invasion of the gut by other strains of bacteria or viruses. The problem is there is no probiotic on the market that supplies bacteroides for the above reasons (that is, these cannot survive outside the human gut for more than a few minutes). If we eat probiotics which have been artificially cultured, for a short while the levels of these probiotics in the gut do increase. However, as soon as we stop eating them, levels taper off and may disappear. Ideally for bacteria to be accepted into the normal gut and remain, they have to be programmed first through somebody else's gut (in this case, mother's).

So, when it comes to repleting gut flora, there are two ways that we can go about this – either we can take probiotics very regularly (and the cheapest way to do this is to grow your own probiotics) or to take bacteroides directly. Indeed, this latter technique is well established in the treatment of *Clostridium difficile* (a normally fatal gastroenteritis in humans) and interestingly in idiopathic (of unknown origin) diarrhoea in horses. In the latter case, horses are inoculated with the bacteria from the gut of another horse. These ideas have been developed further by Dr Thomas Borody with his ideas on faecal bacteriotherapy, which can provide a permanent cure in cases of ulcerative colitis, severe constipation, *Clostridium difficile* infection and pseudomembranous colitis. The reason this technique works so well is because the most abundant bacteria in the large bowel, bacteroides, cannot survive outside the human gut and cannot be given by any other route.

The gut microbiome is extremely stable and difficult to change. Therefore, if you are going to take probiotics, you have to be prepared to take them for the long term. Many preparations on the market are ineffective. Those found to be most effective are those milk ferments and live yoghurts where the product is freshly made. It is not really surprising. Keeping bacteria alive is difficult and it is not surprising that they do not survive dehydration and storage at room temperature. So, your best chance of eating live viable bacteria is to buy live yoghurts or drinks. These can be easily grown at home, just as one would make home-made yoghurt. If you cannot grow easily from a culture, then it suggests that the culture is not active, so this is a good test of what is and is not viable (see Chapter 18).

Sleep

Humans evolved to sleep when it is dark and wake when it is light. Sleep is a form of hibernation when the body shuts down in order to repair damage done through use, to conserve energy and to hide from predators. The normal sleep pattern that evolved in hot climates is to sleep, keep warm and conserve energy during the cold nights and then to sleep again in the afternoons when it is too hot to work and to hide away from the midday sun. As humans migrated away from the Equator, the sleep pattern had to change with the seasons and as the lengths of the days changed.

After the First World War a strain of Spanish 'flu swept through Europe killing 50 million people worldwide. Some people sustained neurological damage and for some this virus wiped out their sleep centre in the brain. This meant they were unable to sleep at all. All these unfortunate people were dead within two weeks, and this was the first solid scientific evidence that sleep was as essential for life as food and water. Indeed, all living creatures require a regular 'sleep' (or period of quiescence) during which time healing and repair take place. You must put as much work into your sleep as your diet. Without a good night's sleep on a regular basis all other interventions are undermined.

Syndrome X

Syndrome X is a pre-diabetic state, also known as 'metabolic syndrome', when blood sugar levels see-saw between too high and too low in the presence of excessively high levels of insulin.

Toxins

Toxins are substances that are dangerous to the body because they inhibit normal metabolism, damage the structure of the body or are wasteful of its resources. Organophosphates, for example, inhibit the essential process of oxidative phosphorylation. Toxic metals can stick onto DNA and trigger cancer; they also stick on to proteins to trigger prion disorders. Products of the fermenting gut require energy and micronutrients for the liver to deal with them. Volatile organic compounds (VOCs) may need methylating to detoxify them, and this is a drain on folic acid and vitamin B12.

Toxins come from the outside world (exogenous) and the inside world (endogenous). Exogenous toxins include POPs (persistent organic pollutants), metals, radiation (most of this comes from the medical profession), toxic halides (fluorides, bromides) and many more. A major source of toxic stress is from prescription medication. Endogenous toxins come from the fermenting gut, natural toxins in foods (e.g. lectins, mycotoxins), breakdown products of normal metabolism, inflammation and other such. Modern Western lifestyles mean we are inevitably exposed to chemicals.

Yeast problems – including Candida

Yeast is one of the common fermenting microbes in the upper gut and is part of the upper fermenting gut issue (see page 217). Yeast problems are an inevitable problem of Western diets, which are high in carbohydrates. The problem is worsened by antibiotics, the Pill and HRT.

Problems may arise initially because yeast numbers build up, sometimes to produce overt infections such as oral thrush, perineal thrush or skin tinea infections (ringworm, athlete's foot, fungal toenails, tinea etc). With chronic exposures there is the potential to sensitise to yeast and that causes much worse problems, characterised by itching, pain and inflammation. Psoriasis may be allergy to yeast; ditto chronic cystitis and interstitial cystitis.

Useful resources and products

1. Ketone breath meter

Many of the Dr Myhill Facebook Group members use these meters:

Nebula Digital Ketone Breathe Analyzer

GDbow Digital Ketone Meter

2. Testing laboratories

No practitioner referral is needed for these:

https://aonm.org

https://medichecks.com

www.mineralstate.com

www.btsireland.com/joomla/

https://smartnutrition.co.uk/health-tests/

https://thriva.co

These laboratories require a practitioner referral:

www.gdx.net/uk

www.doctorsdata.com

www.greatplainslaboratory.com

www.biolab.co.uk

3. Supplement resources

Sunshine Salt from 'Sales at Dr Myhill':

One teaspoon (5 mg) contains all the minerals and vitamin D needed for one day

www.salesatdrymyhill.co.uk/sunshine-salt-300-g-392-p.asp

Vitamins, minerals and herbal supplements

UK www.salesatdrmyhill.co.uk

UK www.biocare.co.uk

UK www.naturesbest.co.uk

USA www.swansonvitamins.com

USA www.purtan.com

Herbs for cooking

UK www.indigo-herbs.co.uk

UK www.hydridherbs.co.uk

USA www.mountainroseherbs.com

4. Exemplar food suppliers

These are some excellent examples. There are many more very good suppliers available also.

Vegan cheese: Bute Island (www.buteisland.com) for vegan cheese

Sauerkraut: Goodness Direct (www.goodnessdirect.co.uk)

Grace Coconut Milk (www.salesatdrmyhill.co.uk/coconut-milk-1-litre-grace-pre-mium-thai-335-p.asp and other good food sites)

COCO Yoghurt (https://cocos-organic.com and other good food sites)

'Coconut Collaborative' Yoghurt (www.waitrose.com/ecom/products/the-coco-nut-collaborative-natural/501386-405600-405601 and other good food sites)

Pork Scratchings (www.amazon.co.uk/Awfully-Posh-Anglesea-Salt-Crackling/dp/B00BPRGJUW/ref=sr_1_1_sspa (just pork rind and salt))

Organic golden linseed: Many of the Dr Myhill Facebook Group members use Suma Organic Golden Linseed (www.amazon.co.uk/Suma-Prepacks-Organic-Linseed-Golden/dp/B01061U62Y/ref=sr_1_6) and there are many other good suppliers

Chocolate:

> Green and Black's organic 85% dark chocolate (www.ocado.com/products/green-black-s-organic-85-dark-34818011 and other good food suppliers)

> Montezuma 100% dark chocolate: This is preferred by many of the Dr Myhill Facebook Group members (www.amazon.co.uk/Montezumas-Absolute-Black-Chocolate-Gluten-free/dp/B0853DVDTW/ref=sr_1_1 and many other good food suppliers)

Beef jerky and biltong (www.jacklinks.online is one good supplier)

Organic vegetable box schemes:

> Soil Association (www.soilassociation.org/organic-living/buyorganic/find-an-organic-box-scheme/)

> www.farmdrop.com/category/fruit-and-veg/fruit-and-veg-bundles

> www.abelandcole.co.uk

> https://organibox.org

> or look for a local farm supplier

5. Exemplar herbal tea suppliers

These are some excellent examples but there are many more very good suppliers available.

Tea Lyra (www.tealyra.co.uk) for herbal teas

Rooibos decaffeinated tea: one example is www.birdandblendtea.com/products/rooibos-matcha-tea

Clipper decaffeinated tea (www.birdandblendtea.com/products/rooibos-matcha-tea)

6. Advice on how to garden organically

Garden Organic: Formerly known as Henry Doubleday Research Association, for advice on how to garden organically whether your garden is large or small go to: www.gardenorganic.org.uk/

References

Chapter 1: Why we should all be eating a Paleo-Ketogenic diet

1. Dawkins R. *The Selfish Gene.* OUP 1976.
2. Gibson G. Staff profile, Food and Nutritional Sciences, University of Reading. www.reading.ac.uk/food/about/staff/g-r-gibson.aspx (accessed 24 June 2021).
2. Berg RD. Bacterial translocation from the gastrointestinal tract. *Adv Exp Med Biol* 1999; 473: 11-30. https://pubmed.ncbi.nlm.nih.gov/10659341/
3. Dr Anthony obit. www.leeds.ac.uk/secretariat/obituaries/2011/anthony_honor.html
4. Rashid T, Wilson C, Ebringer A. The Link between Ankylosing Spondylitis, Crohn's Disease, Klebsiella, and Starch Consumption. *Clin Dev Immunol* 2013; 2013: 872632. doi: 10.1155/2013/872632 www.ncbi.nlm.nih.gov/pmc/articles/PMC3678459/
5. Ebringer A, Rashid T. Rheumatoid arthritis is caused by a Proteus urinary tract infection. *APMIS* 2014; 122(5): 363-368. doi: 10.1111/apm.12154.
6. For those who are interested in learning more about this topic, please see 'Lactose Intolerance by Country' at https://milk.procon.org/lactose-intolerance-by-country/
7. Green J, Cairns BJ, Casabonne D, Wright FL, Reeves G, Beral V. Height and cancer incidence in the Million Women Study: prospective cohort, and meta-analysis of prospective studies of height and total cancer risk. *Lancet Oncol* 2011; 12(8): 785–794. doi: 10.1016/S1470-2045(11)70154-1 www.ncbi.nlm.nih.gov/pmc/articles/PMC3148429/
8. Gerstein HC. Cow's milk exposure and type I diabetes mellitus. A critical overview of the clinical literature. *Diabetes Care* 1994; 17(1): 13-19. doi: 10.2337/diacare.17.1.13. www.ncbi.nlm.nih.gov/pubmed/8112184
9. Virtanen AM, Rasanen L, Ylonen K, et al. Early introduction of dairy products associated with increased risk of IDDM in Finnish children. *Diabetes* 1993; 42(12): 1786-1790.

doi.org/10.2337/diab.42.12.1786. http://diabetes.diabetesjournals.org/content/42/12/1786.

10. Michaëlsson K, Wolk A, Langenskiold S, et al. Milk intake and risk of mortality and fractures in women and men: cohort studies. *Br Med J* 2014; 349. doi.org/10.1136/bmj.g6015
www.bmj.com/content/349/bmj.g6015

11. Moss M, Freed D. The cow and the coronary: epidemiology, biochemistry and immunology. *Int J Cardiol* doi: 10.1016/s0167-5273(02)00201-2
www.ncbi.nlm.nih.gov/pubmed/12559541

Chapter 2: What is the PK diet?

1. Griffith R, Lluberas R, Luhrmann M. Gluttony in England? Long-term change in diet. IFS Briefing Note BN142. Institute of Fiscal Studies November 2013.
www.ifs.org.uk/bns/bn142.pdf

2. Nutrition Security Institute. White Paper: Human Health, the Nutritional Quality of Harvested Food and Sustainable Farming Systems. 2006 U S Senate Document 264 1936
www.biobased.us/NSI_White%20Paper_Web.pdf

3. Safire W. On language: Brits, Tommies, Poms, Limeys & Kippers. *New York Times Magazine* 27 January 1991.
www.nytimes.com/1991/01/27/magazine/on-language-brits-tommies-poms-limeys-kippers.html (accessed 23 June 2021)

Chapter 3: Balancing up the PK diet

1. Cummings JH, Engineer A. Denis Burkitt and the origins of the dietary fibre. *Nutrition Research Reviews* 2018; 31(1): 1-15. doi.org/10.1017/S0954422417000117
www.cambridge.org/core/journals/nutrition-research-reviews/article/denis-burkitt-and-the-origins-of-the-dietary-fibre-hypothesis/1DA569CF06DB93A4FF2DA54629A5D566

2. Baker R. Mathematical modelling in biology. (Dr Ruth Baker's lecture notes.) 2018.
https://courses-archive.maths.ox.ac.uk/node/view_material/52364 (Accessed 22 November 2021)

3. Weston A Price. Broth is beautiful. The Weston A Price Foundation 1 January 2000.
www.westonaprice.org/health-topics/food-features/broth-is-beautiful/

4. Bredesen DE. Reversal of cognitive decline: A novel therapeutic program. *Aging* 2014; 6(9): 707-717.
www.drmyhill.co.uk/drmyhill/images/0/07/Reversal-of-Cognitive-decline-Bredesen.pdf

Chapter 5: Troubleshooting – Diet, detox and die-off reactions

1. Fulgoni VL, Keast DR, Lieberman HR. Trends in intake and sources of caffeine in the diets of US adults: 2001-2010. *Am J Clin Nutr* 2015; 101(5): 1081-1087. doi: 10.3945/ajcn.113.080077. www.ncbi.nlm.nih.gov/pubmed/25832334
2. Cueto E. How old are caffeinated drinks? *Bustle* 16 September 2015. www.bustle.com/articles/110861-how-old-is-coffee-the-first-caffeinated-beverages-might-be-1200-years-old-so-heres-a

Chapter 6: The PK pantry

1. Traditional. Scarborough Fair lyrics. https://genius.com/Traditional-scarborough-fair-lyrics
2. Amy Nuttall. Scarborough Fair. 20 March 2011. www.youtube.com/watch?v=D7YDOhz7jxo
3. Fernandez C. We're not telling porkies… happy pigs oink more! *Daily Mail* 29 June 2016. www.dailymail.co.uk/sciencetech/article-3665092/We-not-telling-porkies-happy-pigs-oink-Animals-grunts-squeals-help-personalities-content-pens.html

Chapter 8: The PK bakery

1. Allaby RG, Peterson GW, Merriwether DA, Fu YB. Evidence of the domestication history of flax (*Linum usitatissimum L.) from genetic diversity of the sad2 locus. Theor Appl Genet* 2005; 112(1): 58-65. www.ncbi.nlm.nih.gov/pubmed/16215731
2. Hirst K. The eight founder crops and the origins of agriculture. Flax Domestication History. Thought.co 31 August 2018. http://archaeology.about.com/od/Domesticated-Plants/fl/Flax-Domestication-History.htm

Chapter 12: PK main courses – stews and roasts

1. Chisholm H (ed). Coriander. *Encyclopædia Britannica.* 7 (11th ed.). Cambridge, UK: Cambridge University Press; 1911: pp 146.

Chapter 13: PK salads, coleslaw and dressings

1. Spence C. Eating with our ears: assessing the importance of the sounds of consumption on our perception and enjoyment of multisensory flavour experiences. *BMC Flavour* 2015; 4: 3.

doi: 10.1186/2044-7248-4-3 https://flavourjournal.biomedcentral.com/articles/10.1186/2044-7248-4-3

Chapter 14: Puddings, sweets and sweeteners

1. Rycerz K, Jaworska-Adamu JE. Effects of aspartame metabolites on astrocytes and neurons. *Folia Neuropathol* 2013; 51(1): 10-17. doi: 10.5114/fn.2013.34191 www.ncbi.nlm.nih.gov/pubmed/23553132

Chapter 16: Herbs and spices

1. Ingraham C. *Animal Self-medication.* www.carolineingraham.com/store/books/animal-self-medication/
2. Biser JA. Really wild remedies – medicinal plant use by animals. *Zoogoer* Jan-Feb 1998. https://web.archive.org/web/20040630010109/http://nationalzoo.si.edu/Publications/Zoogoer/1998/1/reallywildremedies.cfm
3. Buettner D. The island where people forget to die. *Readers' Digest* 6 April 2016. www.rd.com/article/island-people-forget-to-die/

Chapter 17: PK salt – Sunshine salt

1. http://penelope.uchicago.edu/Thayer/L/Roman/Texts/Pliny_the_Elder/31*.html
2. Eisenberg MJ. Magnesium deficiency and sudden death. *Am Heart J* 1992; 124(2): 544-549. doi: 10.1016/0002-8703(92)90633-7.
3. Mayer A-M. Historical changes in the mineral content of fruits and vegetables. *British Food Journal* 1997; 99(6): 207-211. doi.org/10.1108/00070709710181540 www.emeraldinsight.com/doi/pdfplus/10.1108/00070709710181540

Chapter 18: Fermented foods

1. World Health Statistics 2016: Monitoring health for the SDGs Annex B: tables of health statistics by country, WHO region and globally. World Health Organization. 2016. www.who.int/gho/publications/world_health_statistics/2016/EN_WHS2016_AnnexB.pdf?ua=1
2. Thomas Jefferson to Thomas Cooper, 10 July 1812. http://founders.archives.gov/documents/Jefferson/03-05-02-0179

Chapter 19: PK water

1. Buck B. Don't drink the (warm) water left in a plastic bottle UF/IFAS study says. UF/IFAS. 22 September 2014. http://blogs.ifas.ufl.edu/news/2014/09/22/dont-drink-the-warm-water-ufifas-study-says/

Chapter 22: The carnivore diet

1. McClellan WS, Du Bois EF. Clinical calorimetry: XLV prolonged meat diets with study of kidney function and ketosis. *Journal of Biological Chemistry* 1930; 87(3): 651-668. www.sciencedirect.com/science/article/pii/S0021925818768427
2. Mansfield J. *Arthritis: Allergy, Nutrition and the Environment.* Thorsons; 1995.
3. Darlington LG, Ramsey NW, Mansfield JR. Placebo-controlled, blind study of dietary manipulation therapy in rheumatoid arthritis. *Lancet* 1986; 1(8475): 236-238. doi: 10.1016/s0140-6736(86)90774-9.

Chapter 23: Fasting – a great therapeutic tool

1. Bredesen DE. Reversal of cognitive decline: A novel therapeutic program. *Aging* 2014; 6(9): 707-717. doi: 10.18632/aging.100690 www.ncbi.nlm.nih.gov/pmc/articles/PMC4221920/

Chapter 24: Easy weight loss with the PK diet

1. ASMDS. Estimate of bariatric surgery numbers, 2011-2019. American Society for Metabolic and Bariatric Surgery. March 2021 https://asmbs.org/resources/estimate-of-bariatric-surgery-numbers

Index

Index